Christmas
Adult Coloring Book for Stress Relief

35 Christmas Inspired Designs for Relief from
Stress, Anxiety & Depression

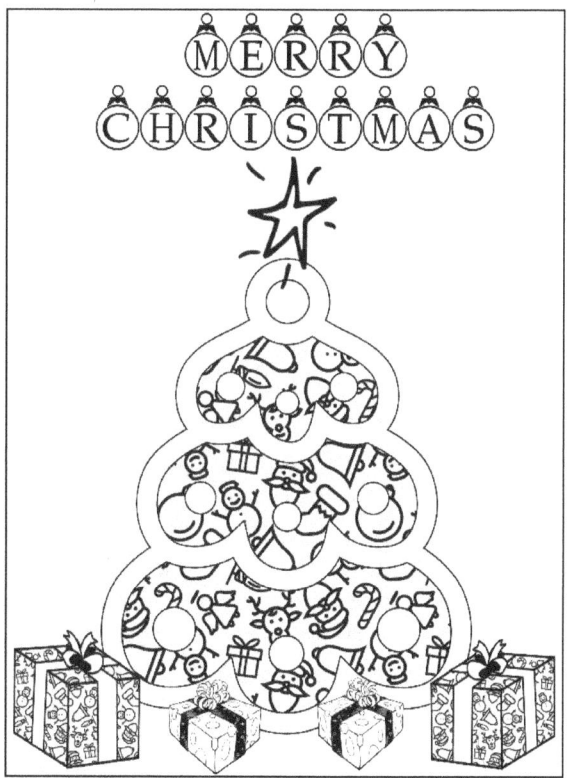

Cover and Book Design by Nerine Martin

Copyright © 2016 Nerine Martin. All rights reserved.

www.ColorYourWayToHappy.com

No part of this book may be reproduced, copied or scanned except for your own personal use and enjoyment.
You may share only the images that you have colored on social media, as long as you attribute
Nerine Martin and include the book name in your post.
These images, either colored or non-colored may not be resold.

ISBN 978-1540694805

A message from Nerine.....

Congratulations on your purchase of *'Christmas Adult Coloring Book for Stress Relief'* and thank you for choosing my coloring book.

The Christmas Holiday season is a wonderful time of the year when many families and friends come together to celebrate. However, it can also be a stressful time for some, especially if you already suffer from conditions such as stress, anxiety and depression.

Inside this beautifully designed 'Christmas Adult Coloring Book' you will find 35 unique Christmas inspired designs that the whole family can come together on Christmas Day to color.

If, like me, you are hosting a festive meal for your family and friends and you know leading up to the day with all the preparation, that this can make you feel a bit anxious, why not take some time for yourself to breathe and relax by coloring a few pages from this book.

It has been proven that using coloring as a form of art therapy, can help relieve symptoms by distracting the mind's thought processes and can also aid as a coping strategy to get through the difficult times.

Use your imagination to make these holiday designs come alive with color, using colored pencils, felt tip markers, gel pens, fluoro markers, metallic pens or crayons. To help prevent any bleed through when using felt tip markers – place a blank sheet of paper behind the page when coloring. You will find spare pages at the back of this book you can tear out and use.

Please remember that your purchase of this Christmas inspired coloring book is for your personal use only and you may not share or copy the uncolored pages for others. Please direct other people to purchase their own, or consider giving them a copy as a lovely Christmas gift. By doing so, you are supporting my art so I can continue to make more coloring books and I thank you for your understanding and support. ☺

In the back of this coloring book you will also find a BONUS of coloring page designs from all of my mindfulness series of adult coloring books published so far.

I truly hope through coloring these designs, my coloring book can make a difference to how you are feeling, and that it can bring some calm to your life as you color. My wish is to help other people just like you, through my coloring books, so that YOU are in total control of your life, not the anxiety, stress or depression!

I wish you and your family a wonderful, safe and peaceful festive season and I hope you enjoy coloring my Christmas book that I absolutely had so much fun creating for you!

Merry Christmas
Nerine ☺

Have you subscribed to my weekly newsletter yet?

All you need to do is go to www.ColorYourWayToHappy.com/freebie and enter your name and email to start receiving my weekly newsletter and you'll also receive a FREE coloring book to print at home!

What customers have to say about the 'COLOR YOUR WAY TO HAPPY' Series of Adult Coloring Books........

"Your mandalas are the most beautiful I've seen anywhere and super gorgeous with the black backgrounds. I want to encourage everyone in this group to order a copy….. Nerine's designs are different from any others you've seen, and they are featured in Adult Coloring Book Treasury 1 and 2" – Shela W.

"I got the mandala volume one and am having a ball with it.
Mandala addicts like me, it is a must have!" – Nessa

"Thank you for drawing beautiful pieces that I can put color to.
Coloring is my sanity, your pieces are calming and relaxing to color" – Christina

"Just Wonderful. Love this book! Can spend hours losing yourself in the mandala designs! Very calming and a great way to de-stress!" – Natalatalie

"…I love the story about this artist and why she did this series of books" – PINPOP

'This series of coloring books is fantastic! Nerine has done such a variety of mandalas in all three books that you get enjoyment/relaxation from each and every one. The paper they are printed on is amazing as well and makes the coloring experience even better. Thank you for producing such a great product.' – Amazon Customer

"I'm really enjoying volume 1…" – Emma

"I received these yesterday and OMG they're beyond awesome! Thank you heaps…" – Chelle

"Thank you for creating such an awesome coloring book with black backgrounds.
They are my favorite!" – Shela

"Beautiful Mandalas! If you just love mandalas, or want to destress this book will help with that. I love this series of coloring book each one is different in the presentation of the mandalas" – PINPOP

"One Mandala a day – great idea!" – Shelly

'Fantastic book for not just anxiety, but will help calm you down from whatever issues are getting to you. Step back, color a bit, and you will be able to focus better.
After coloring, reading the words and thinking, I felt much better.' - Connie

Use This Area To Test Your Colors

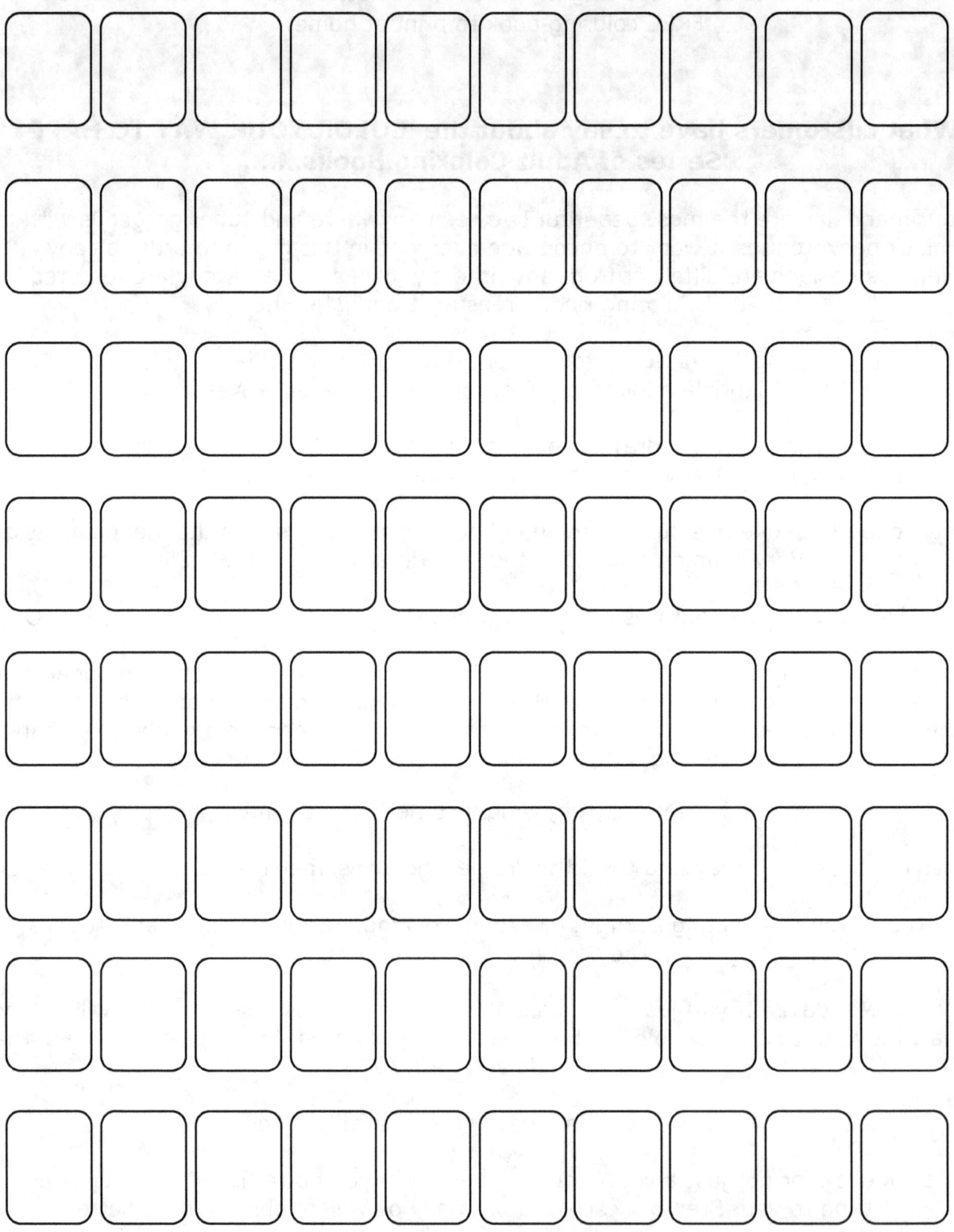

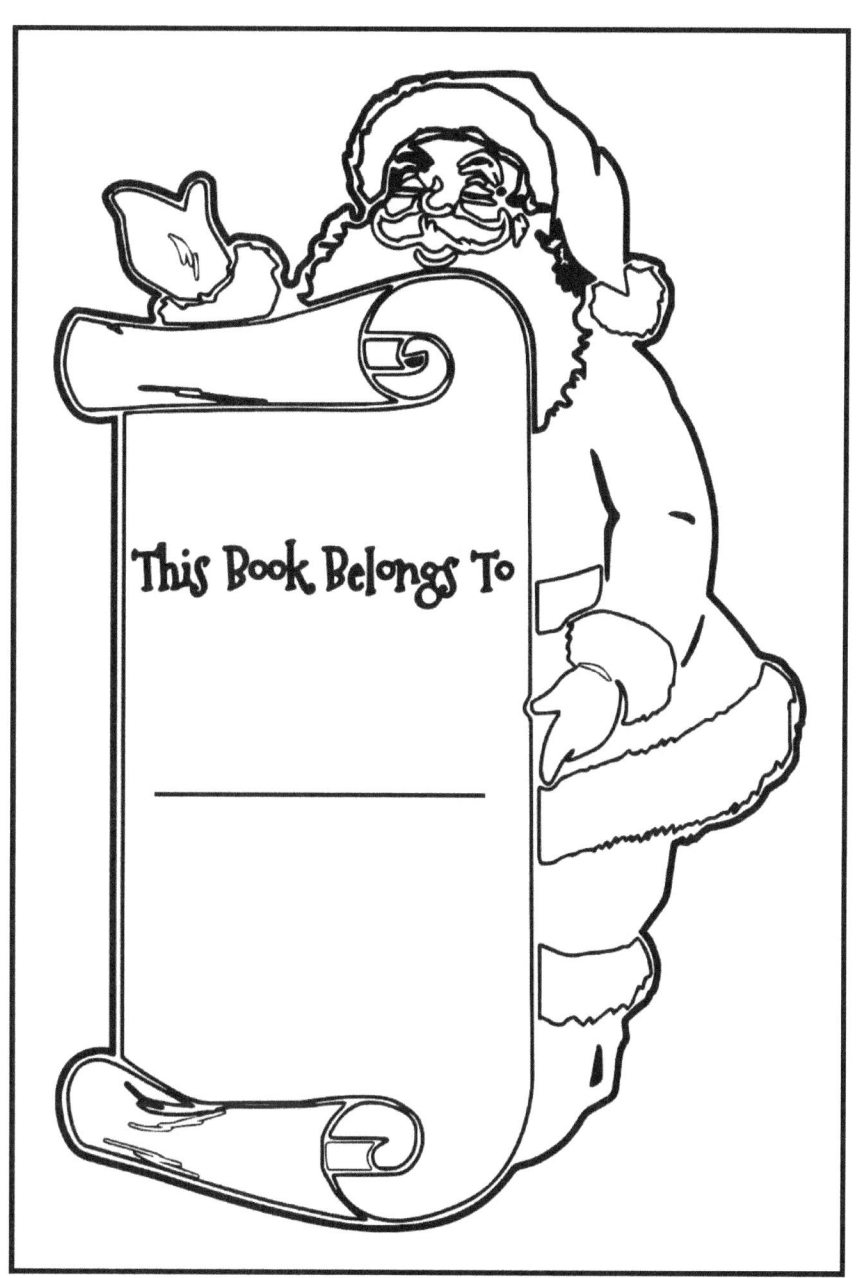

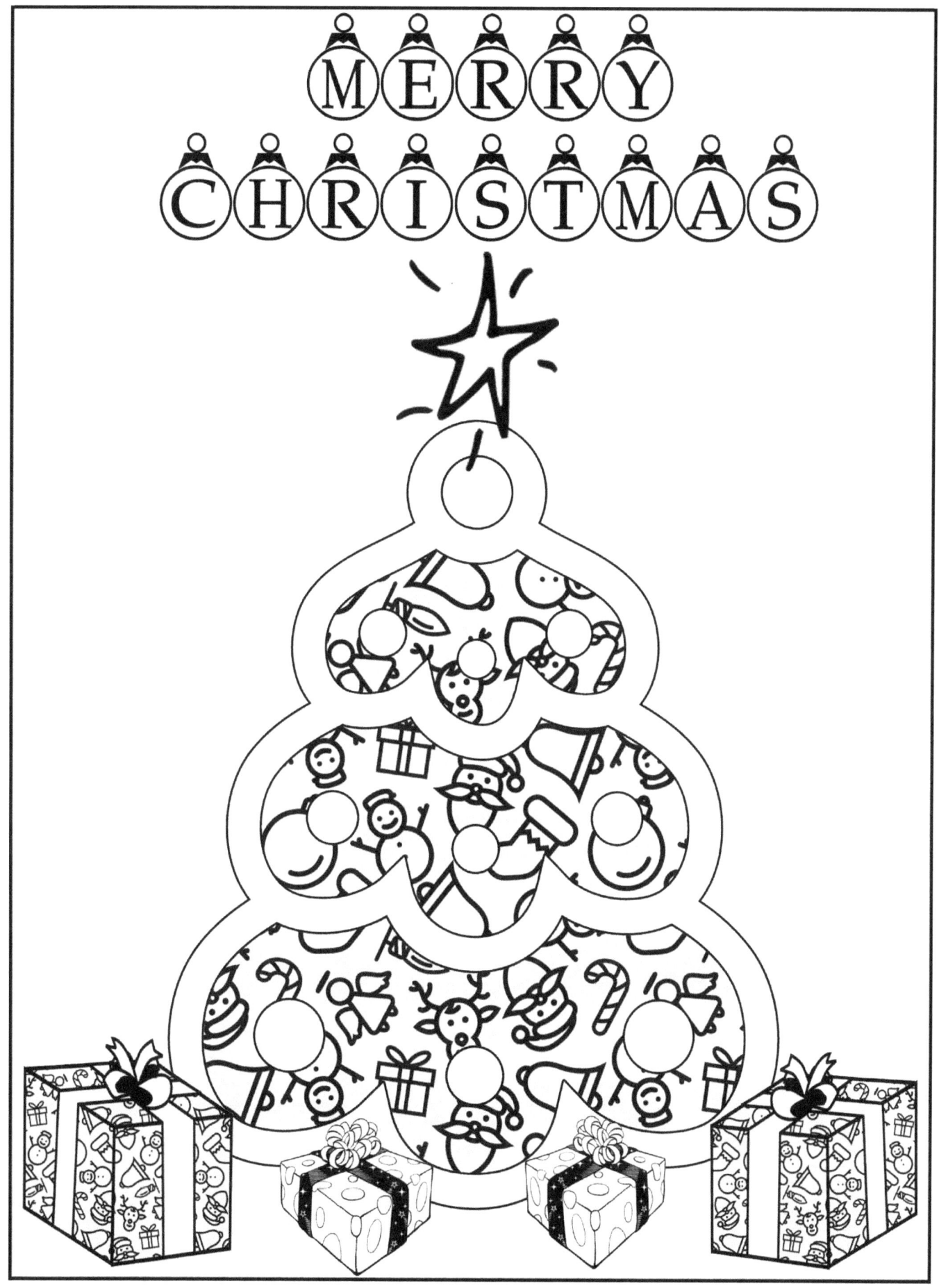

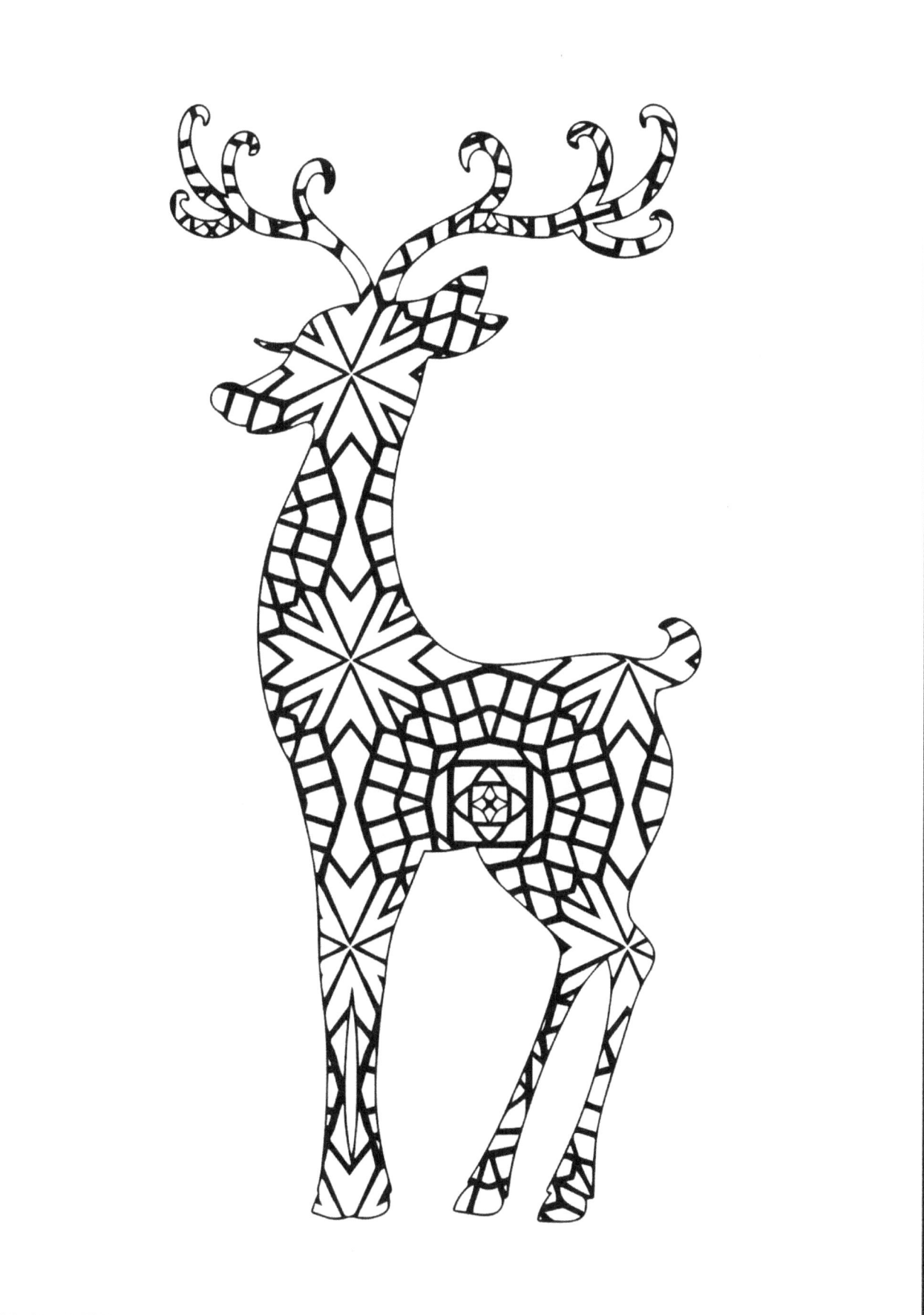

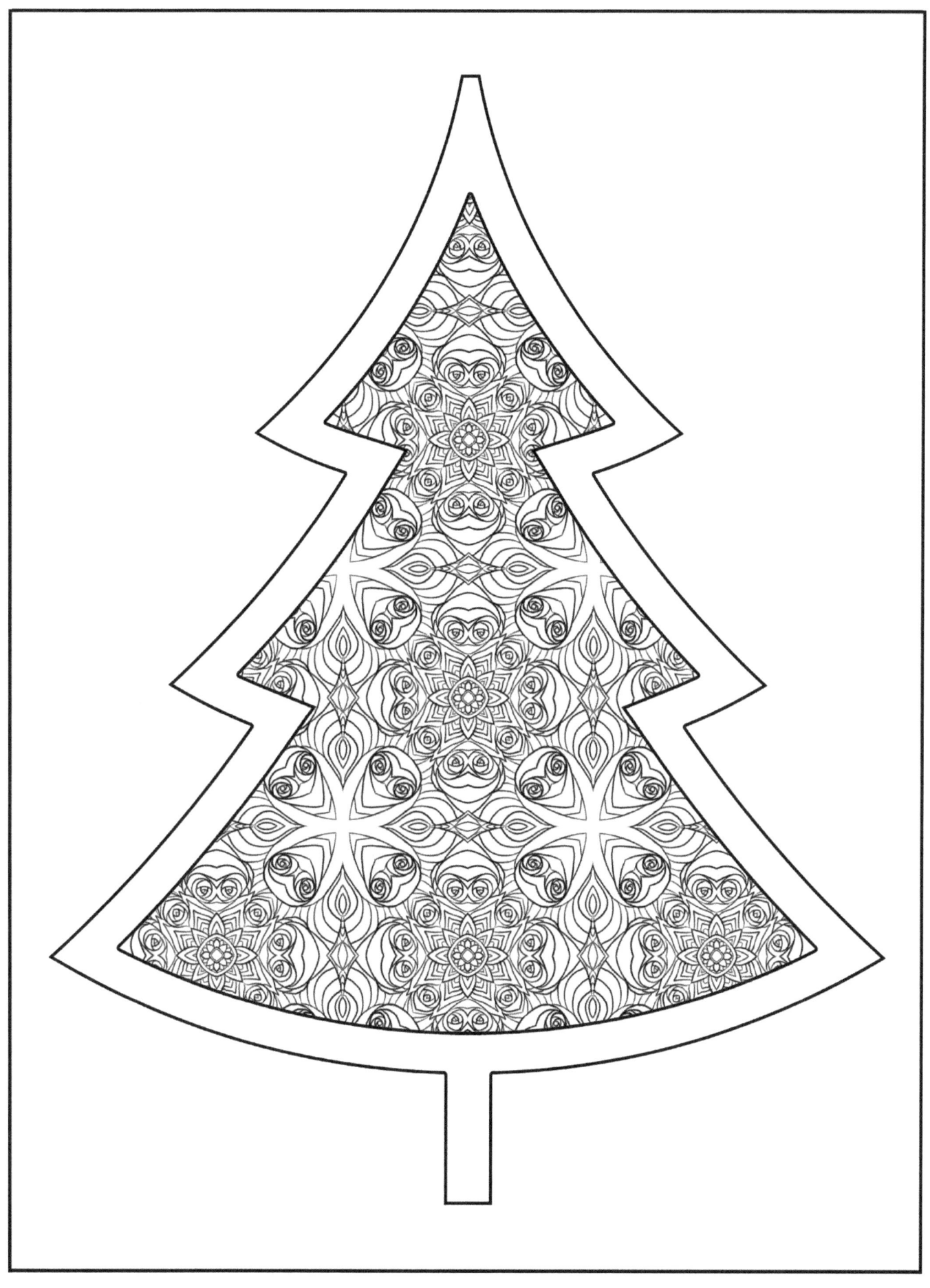

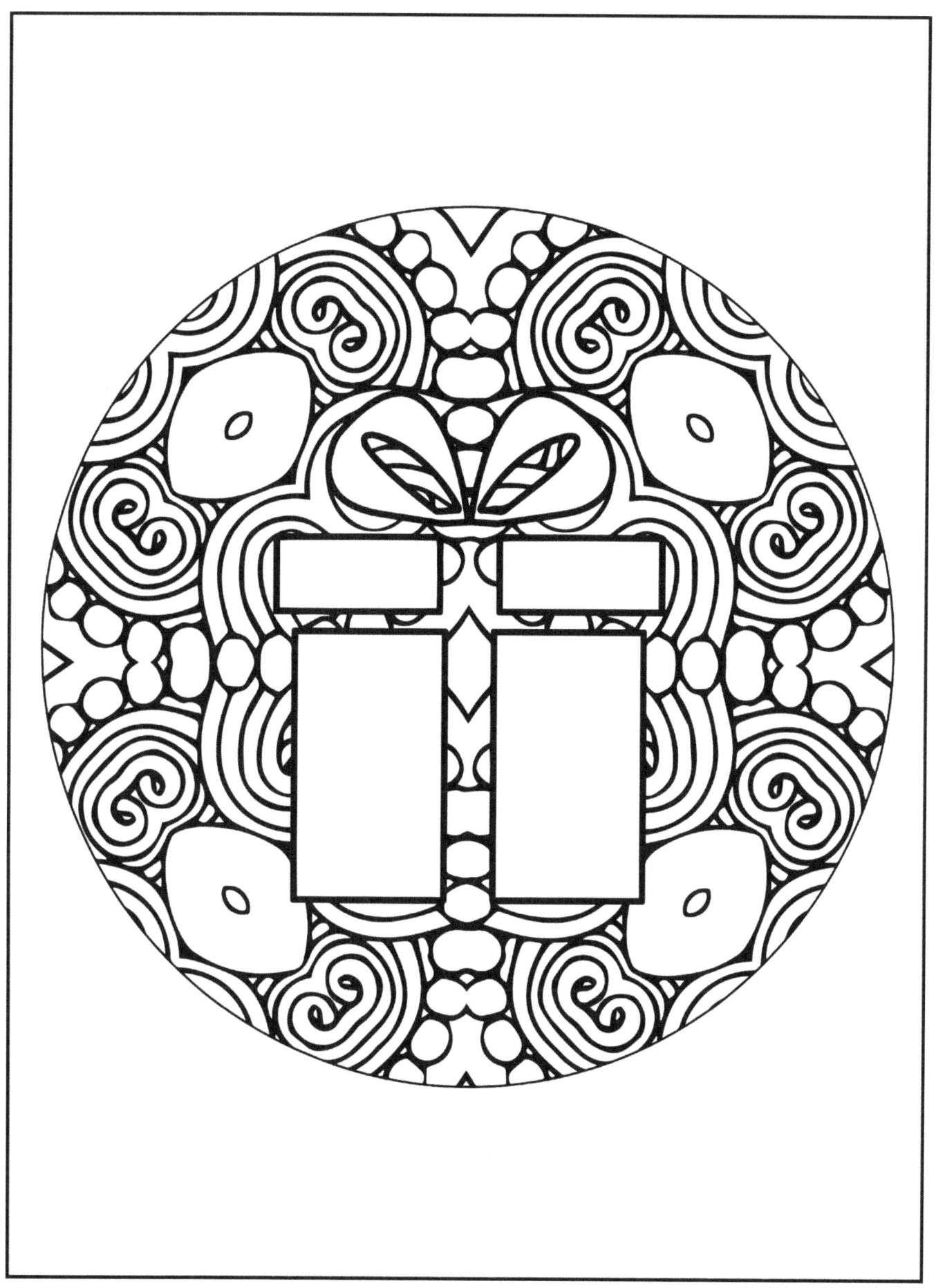

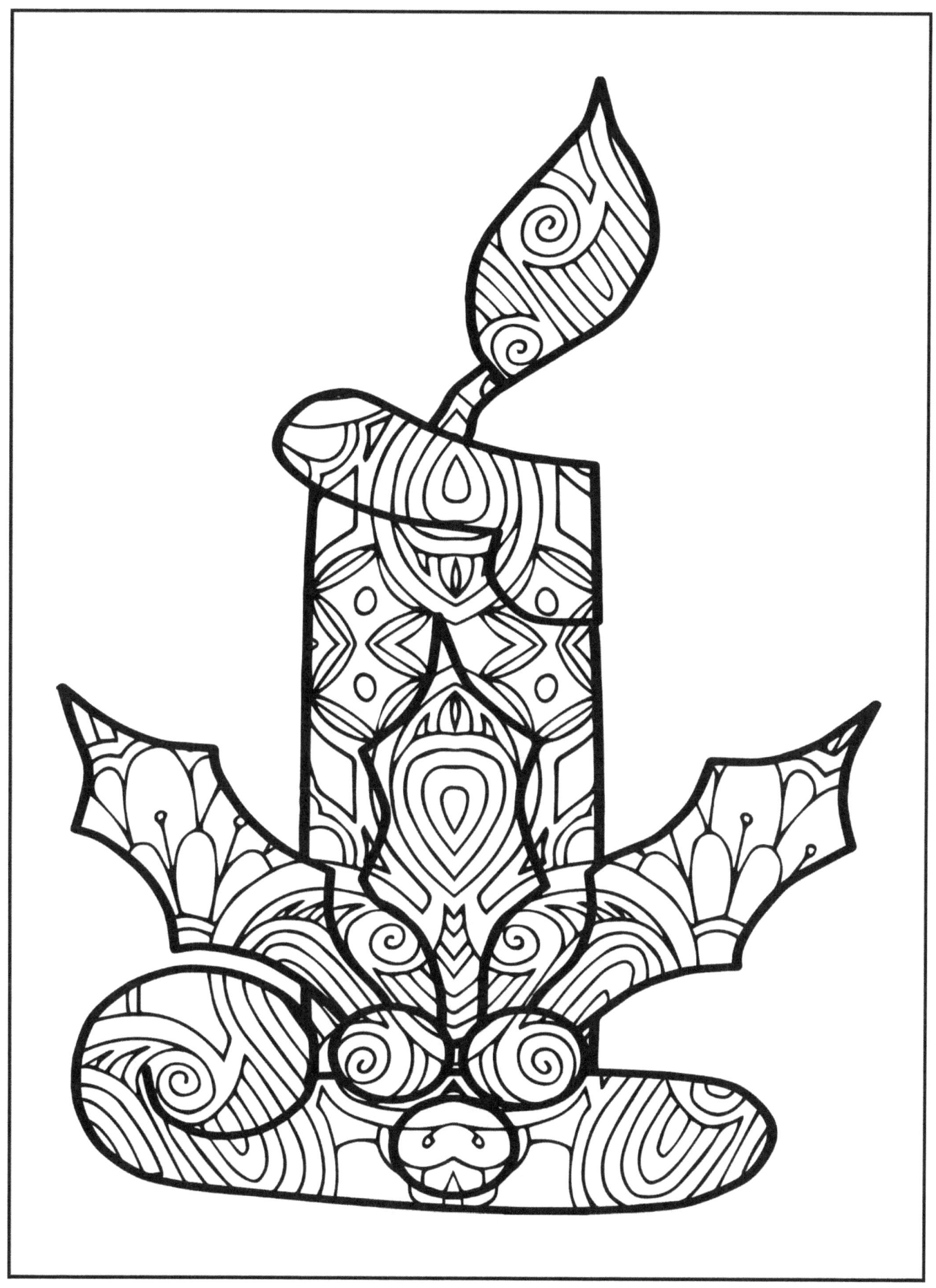

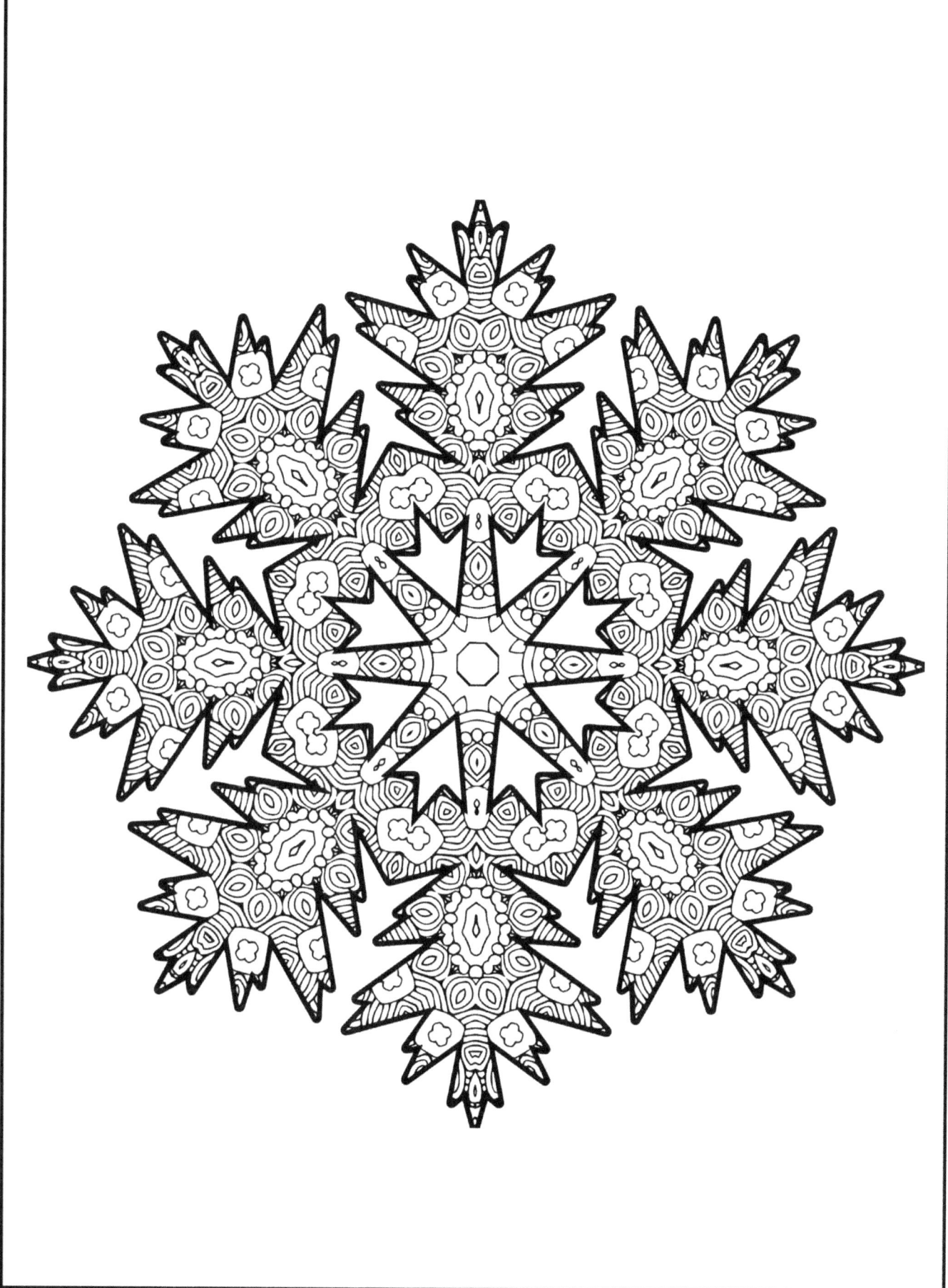

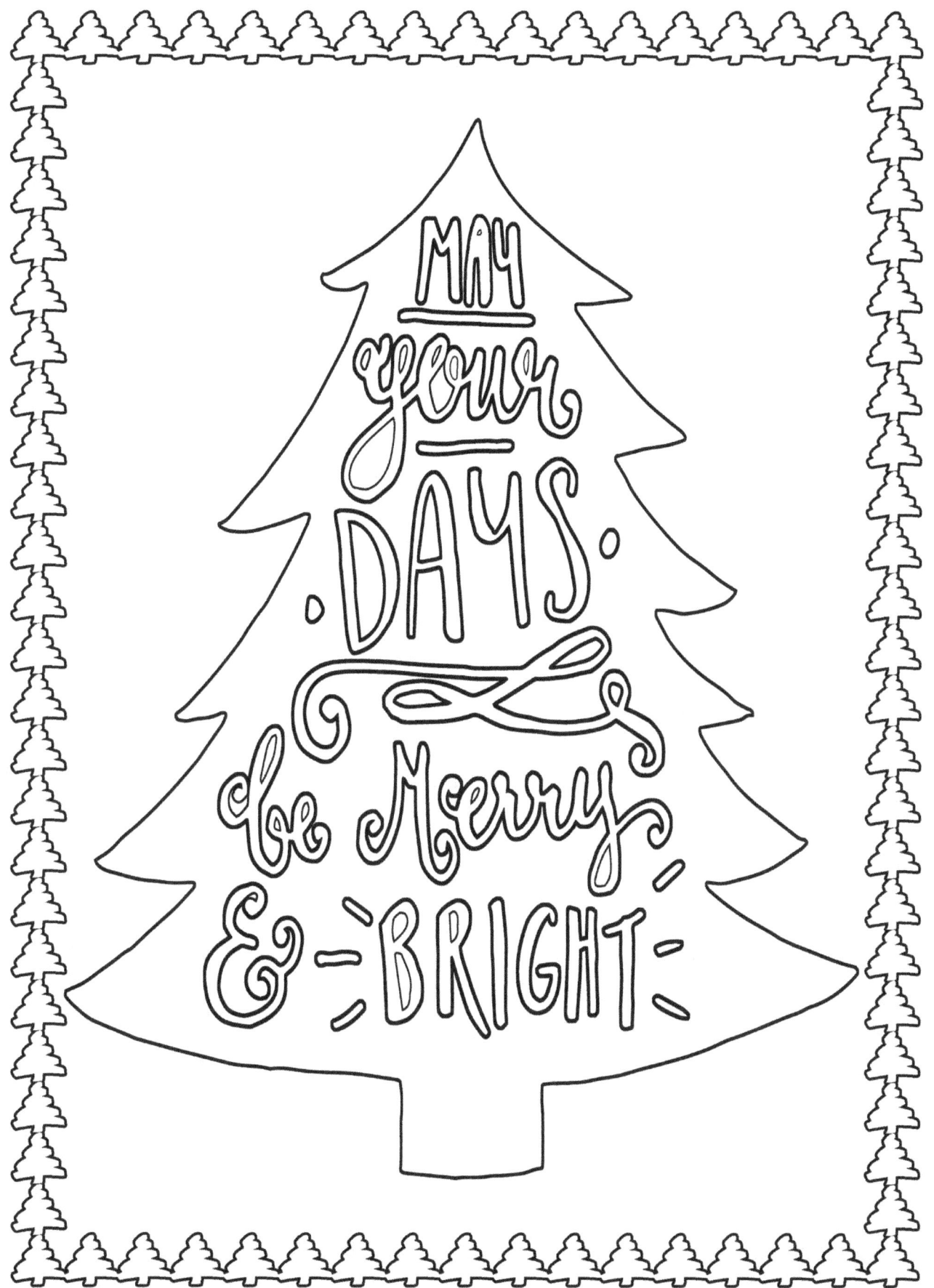

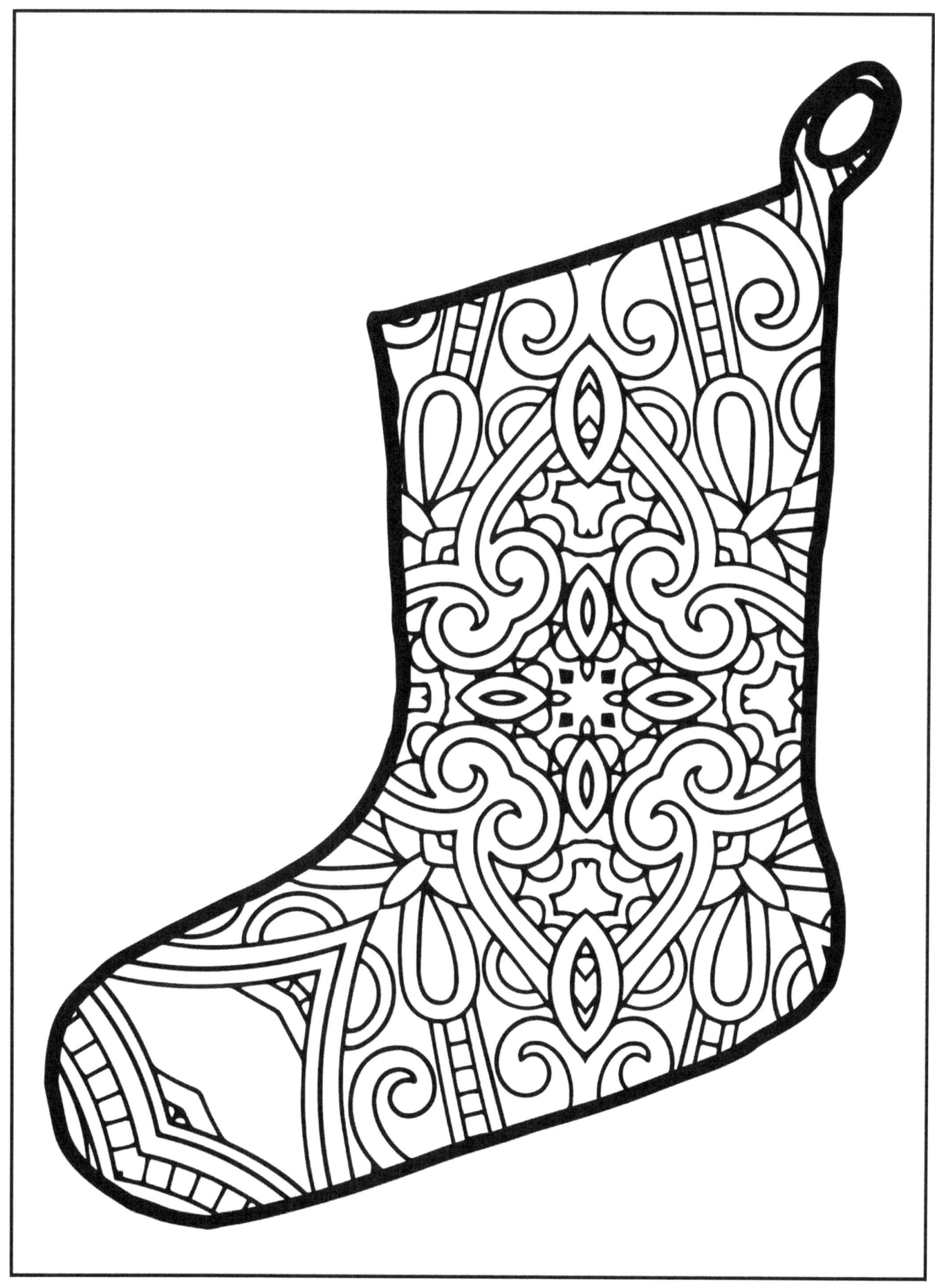

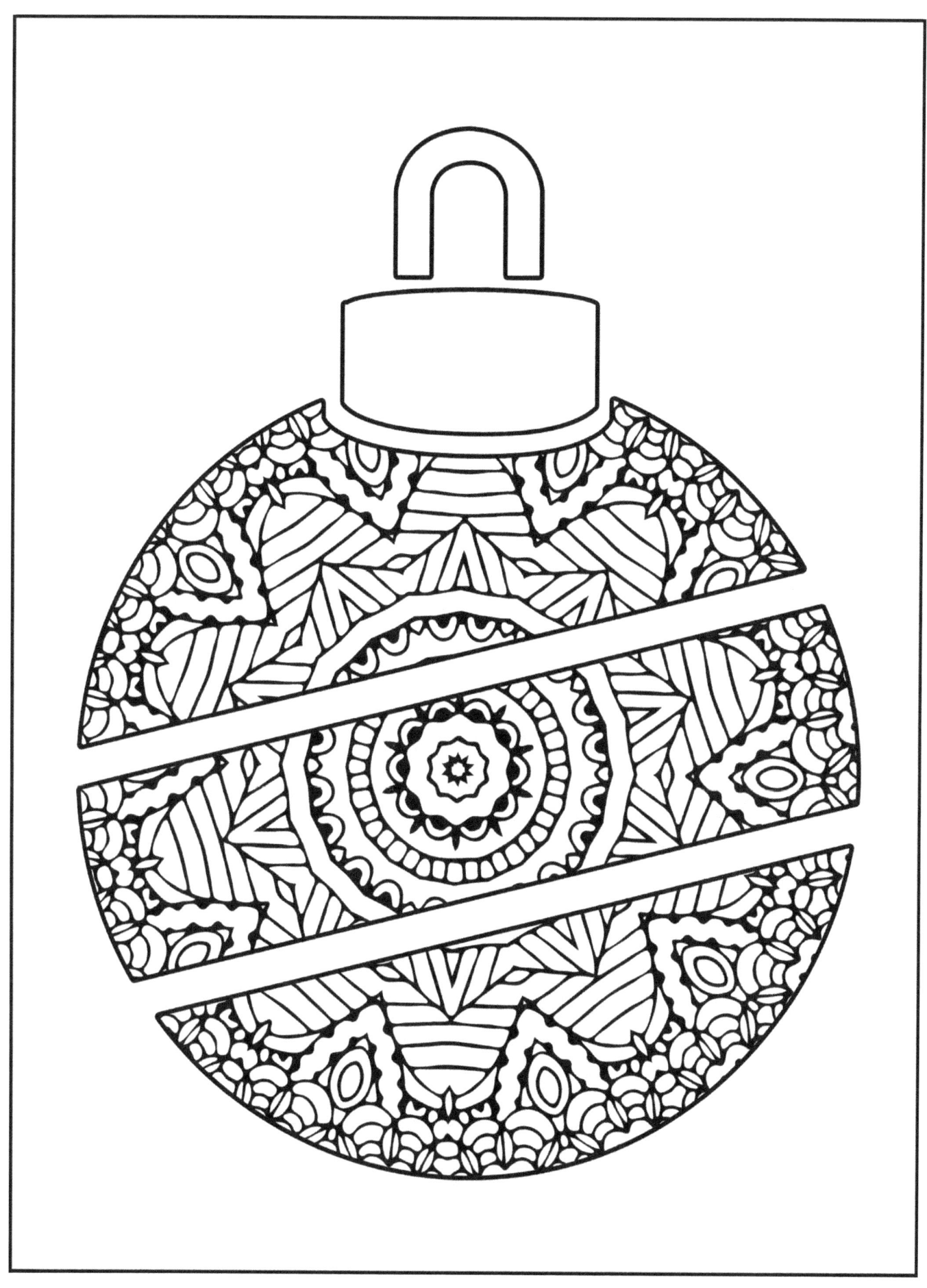

Jingle Bells

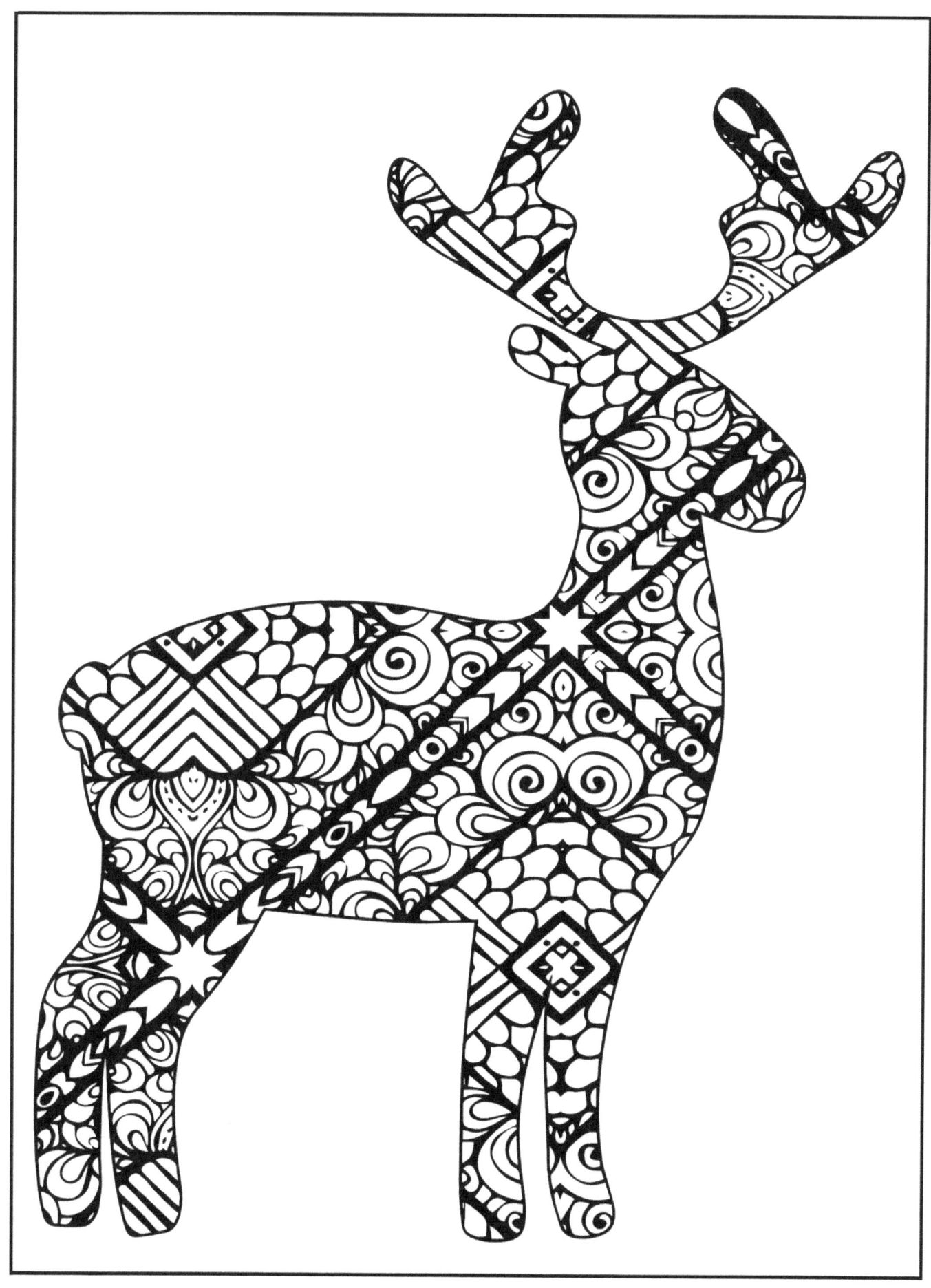

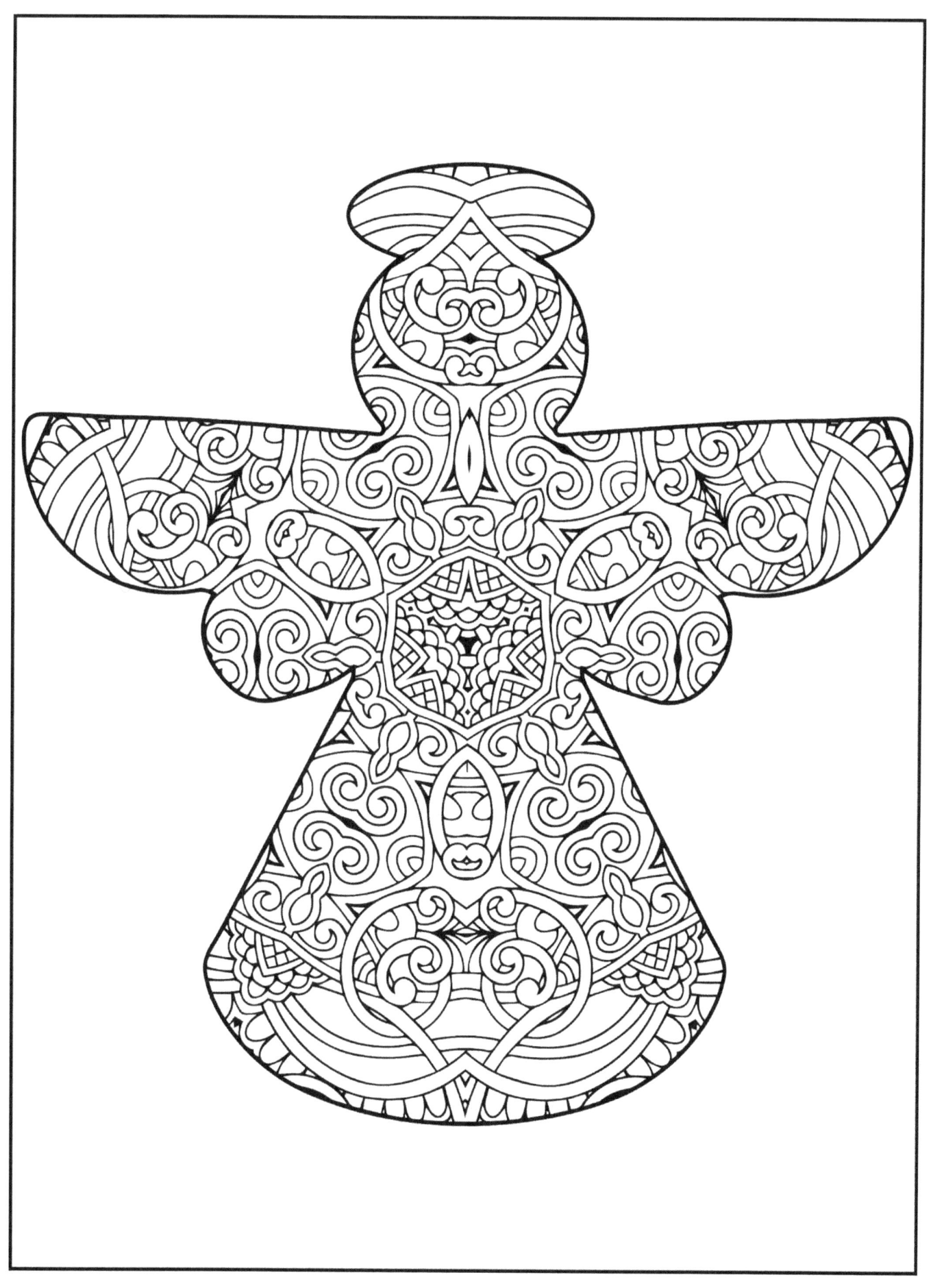

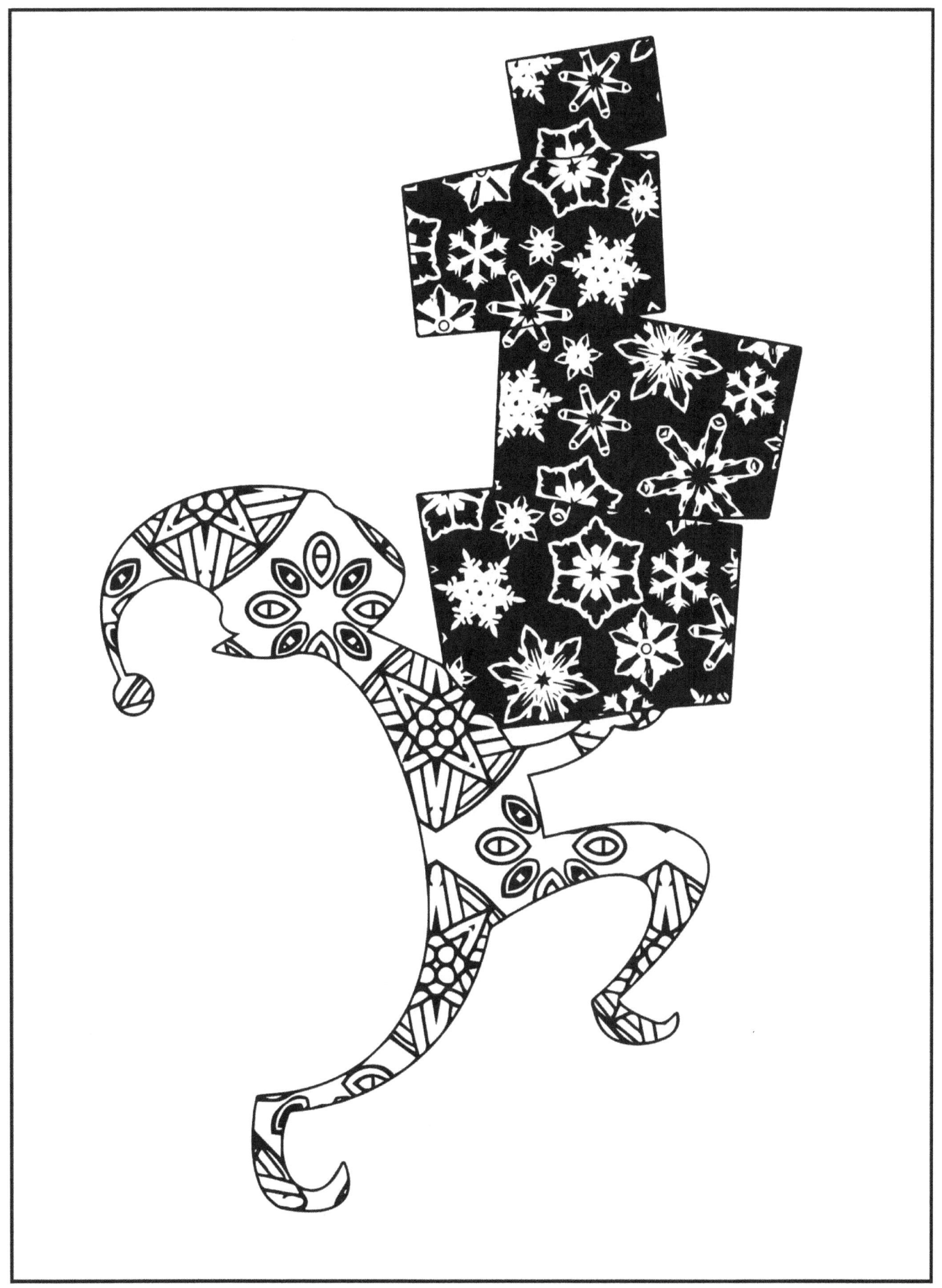

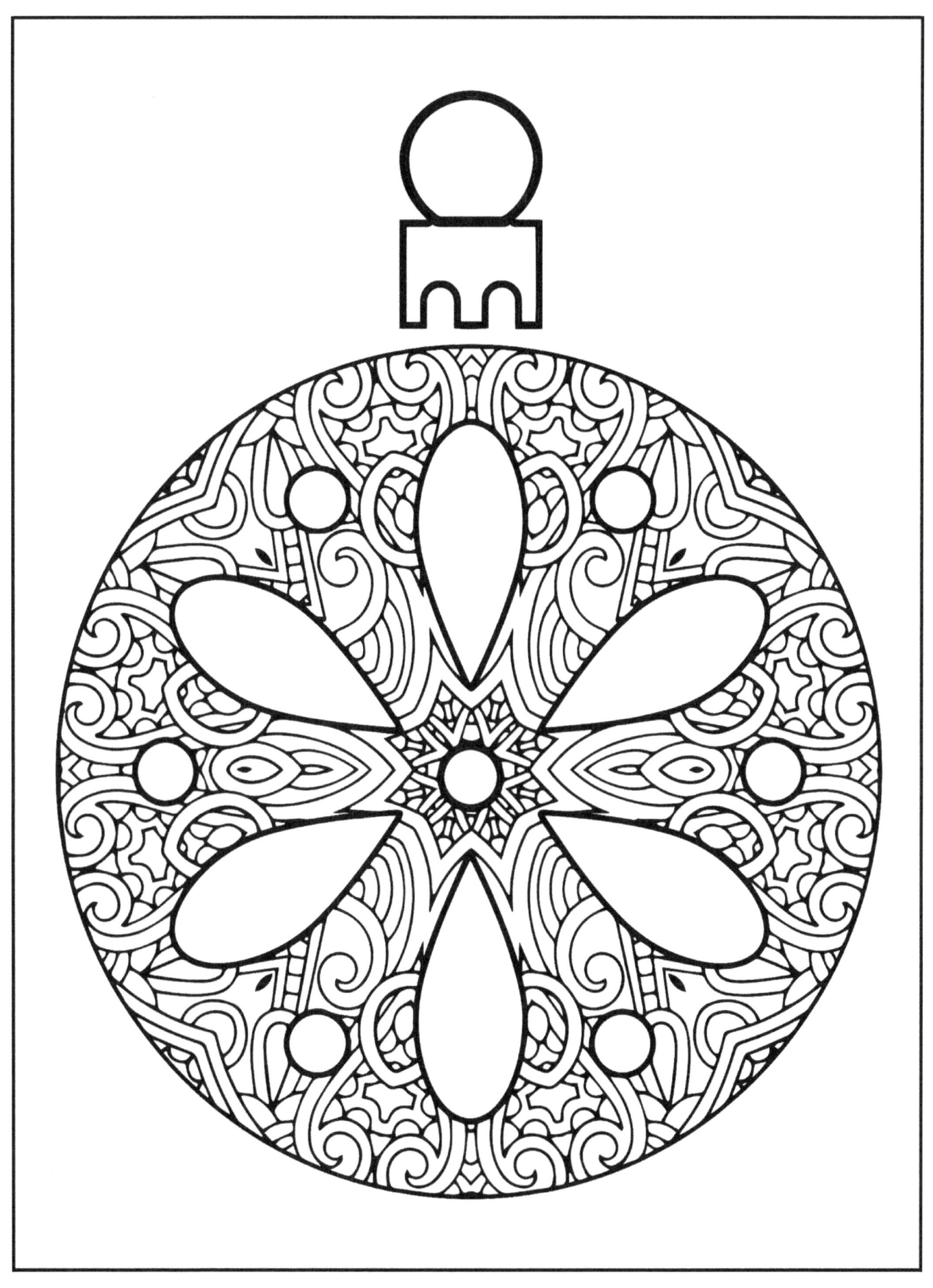

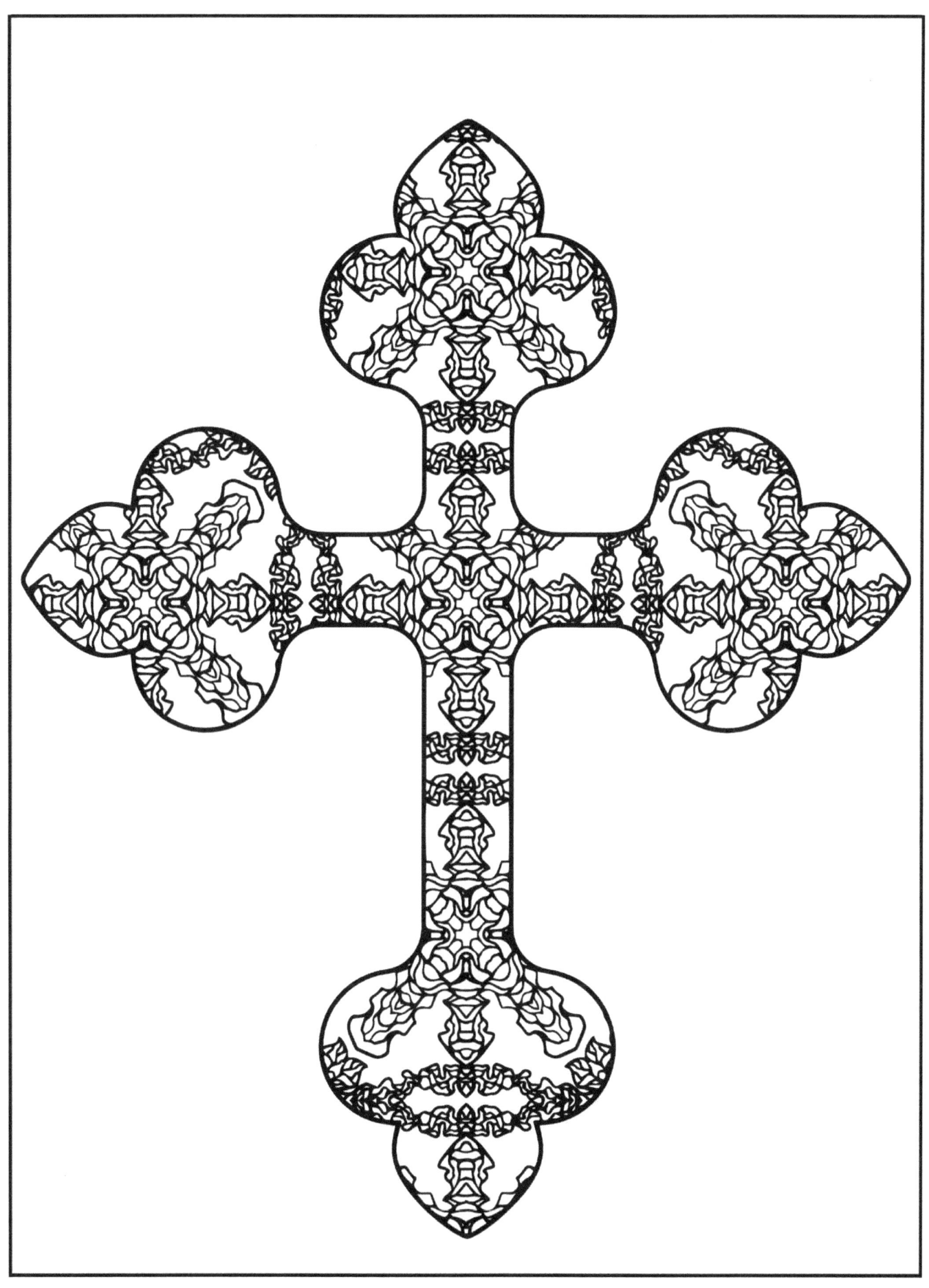

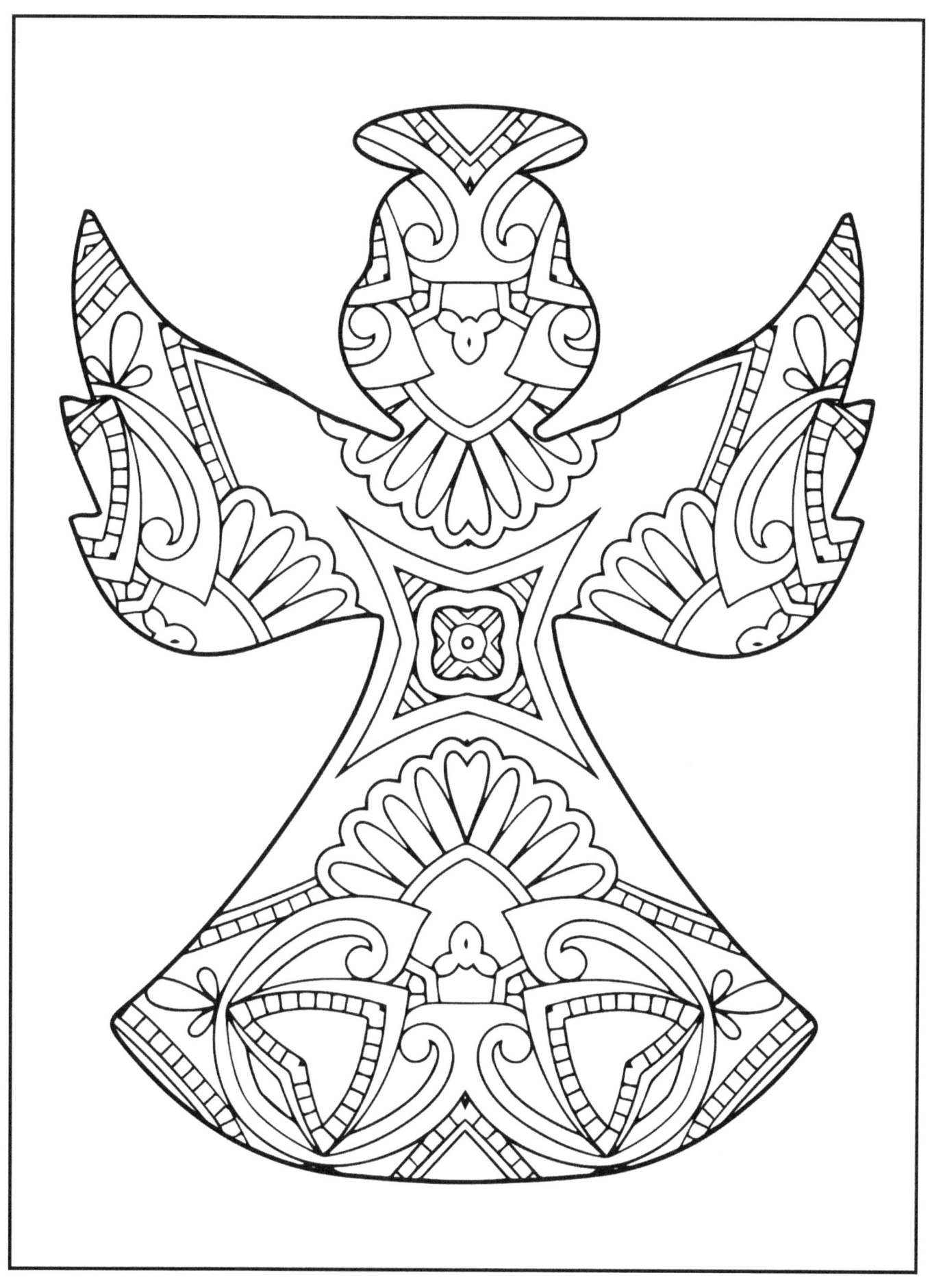

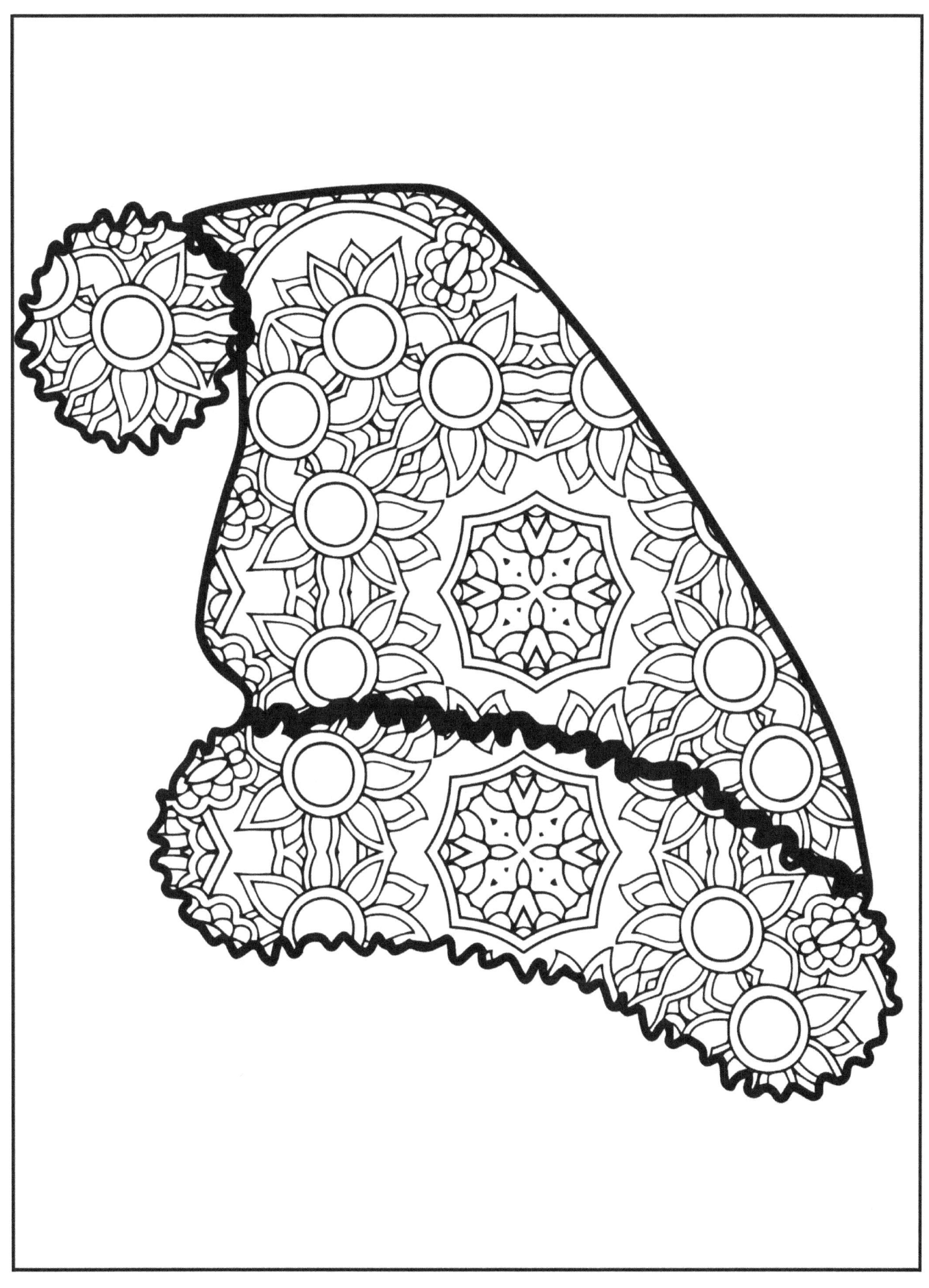

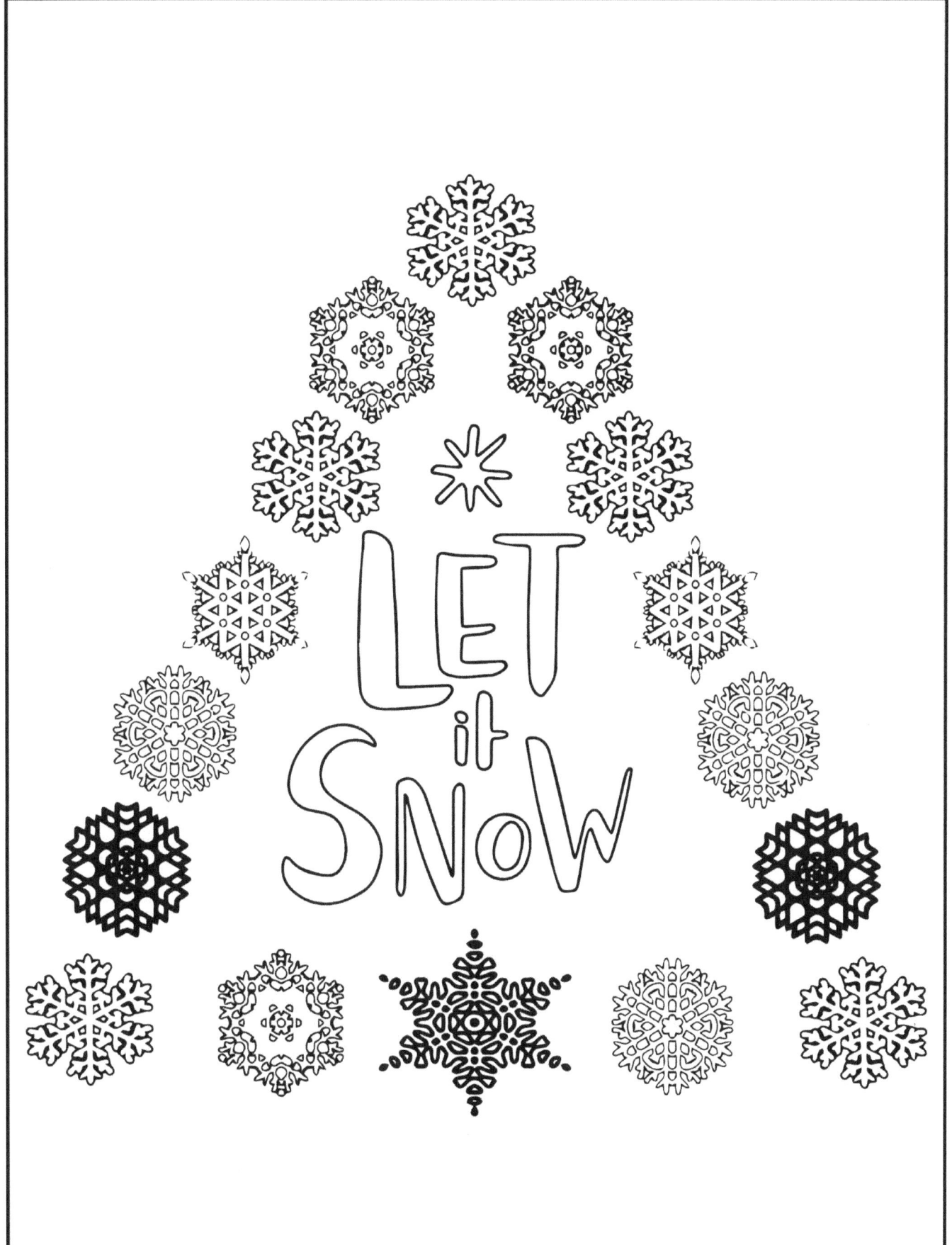

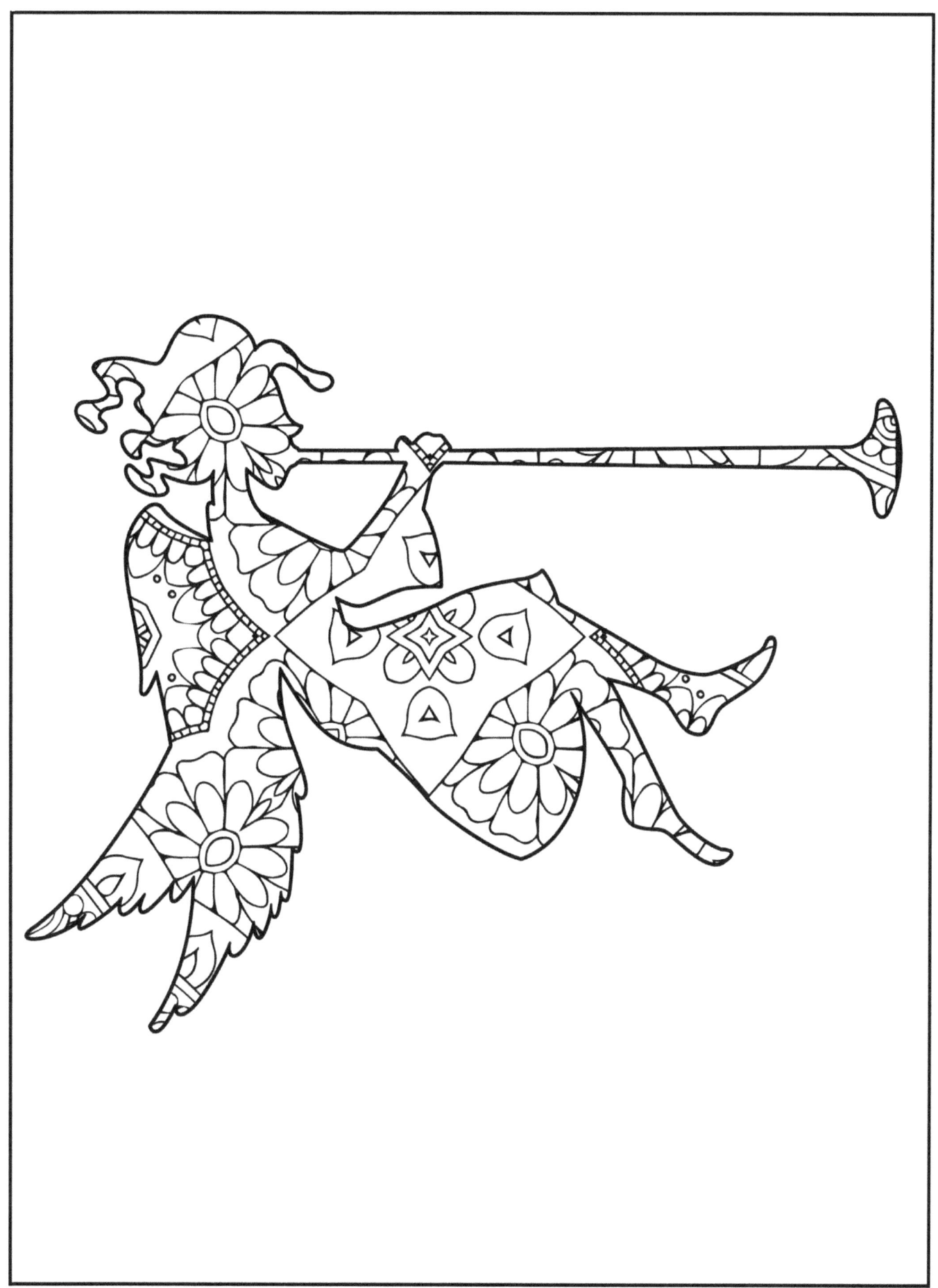

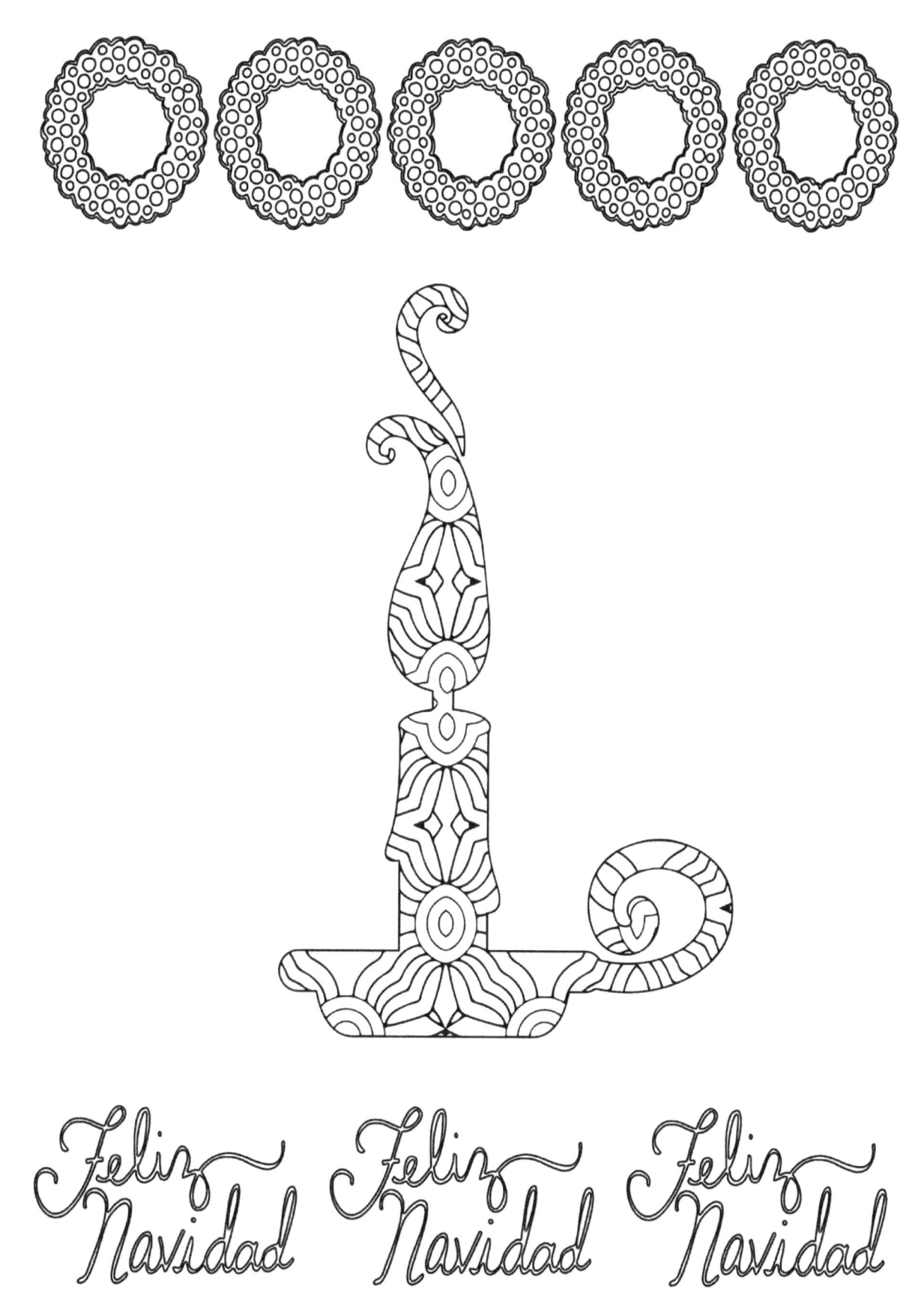

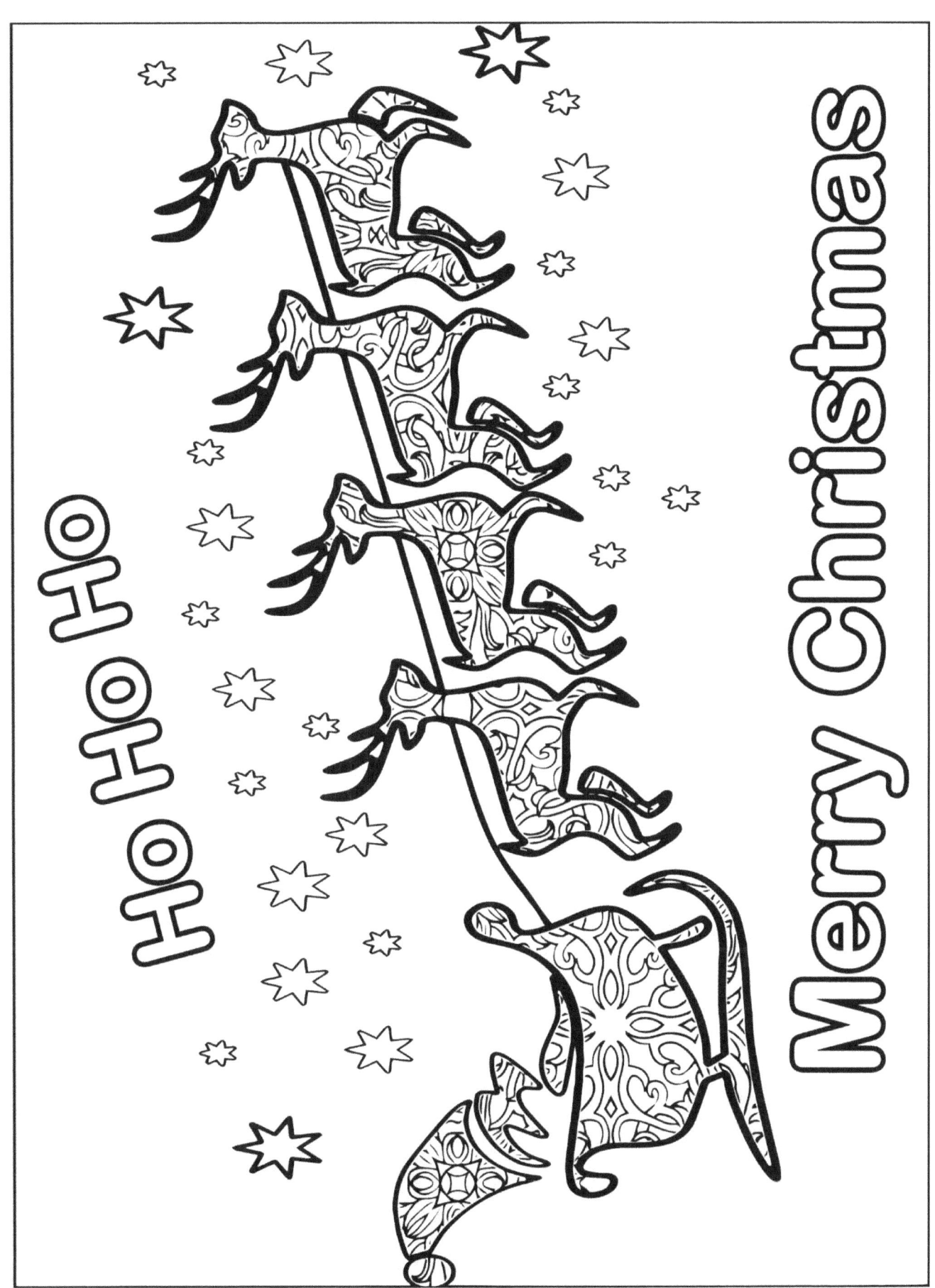

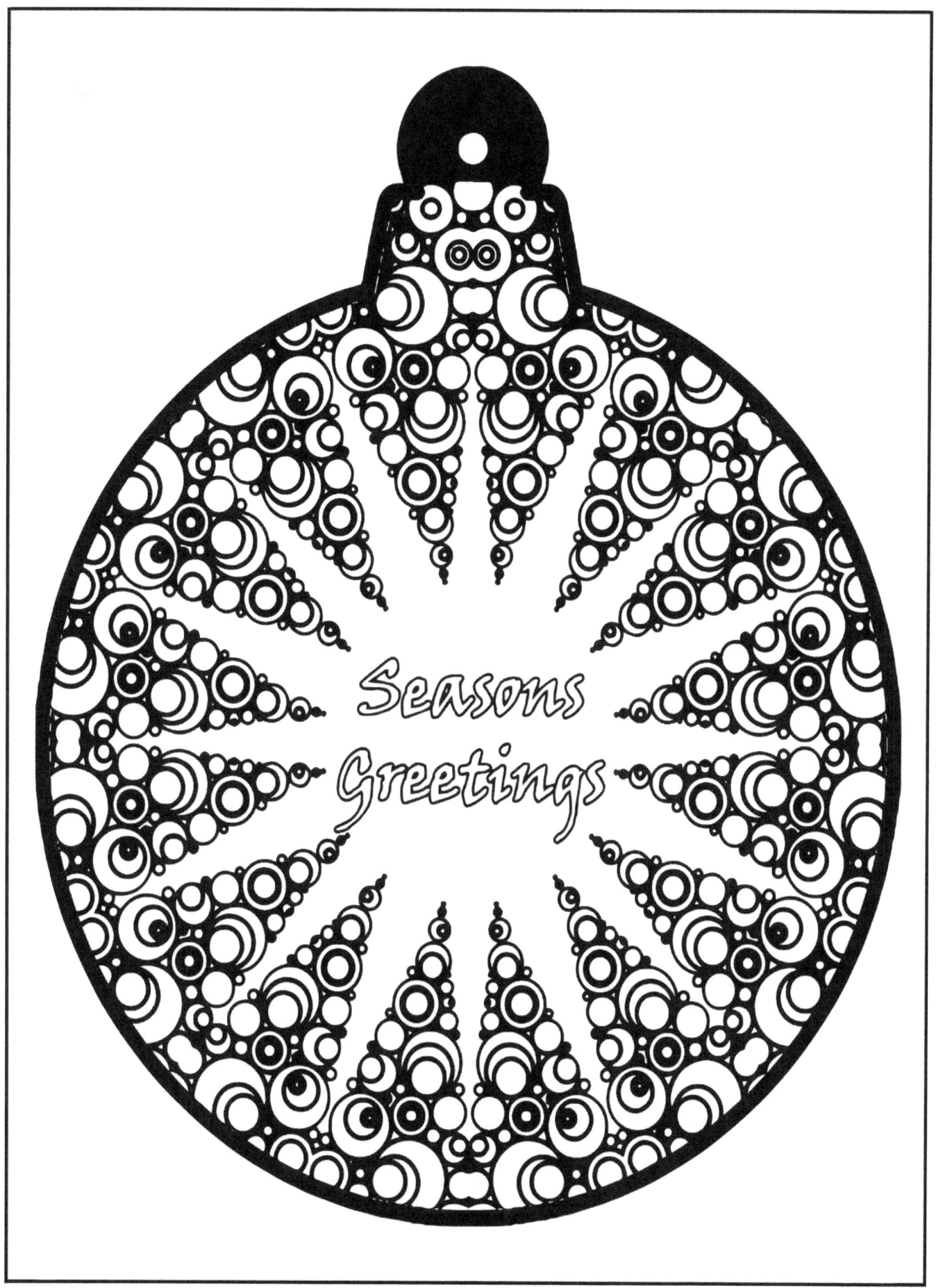

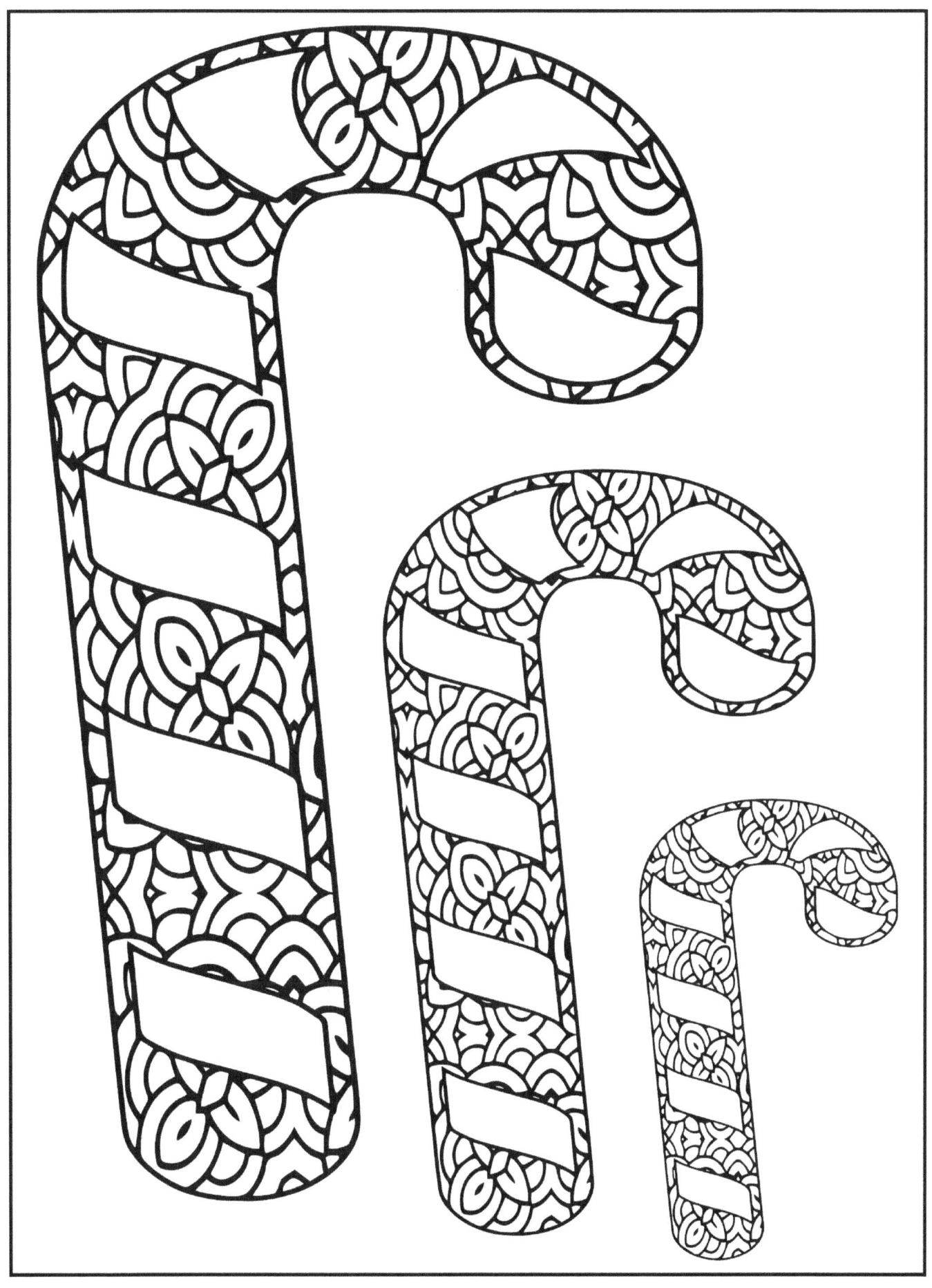

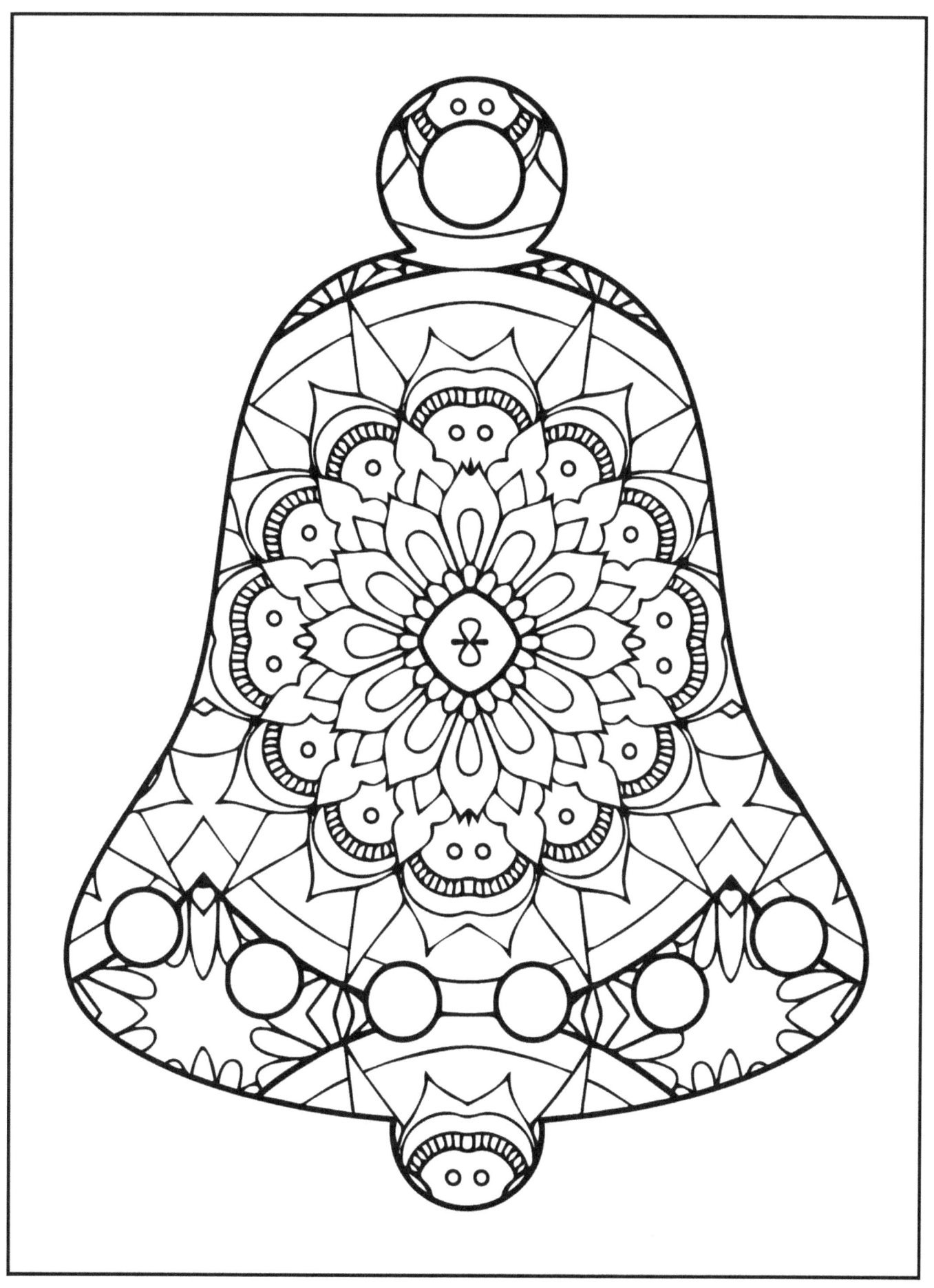

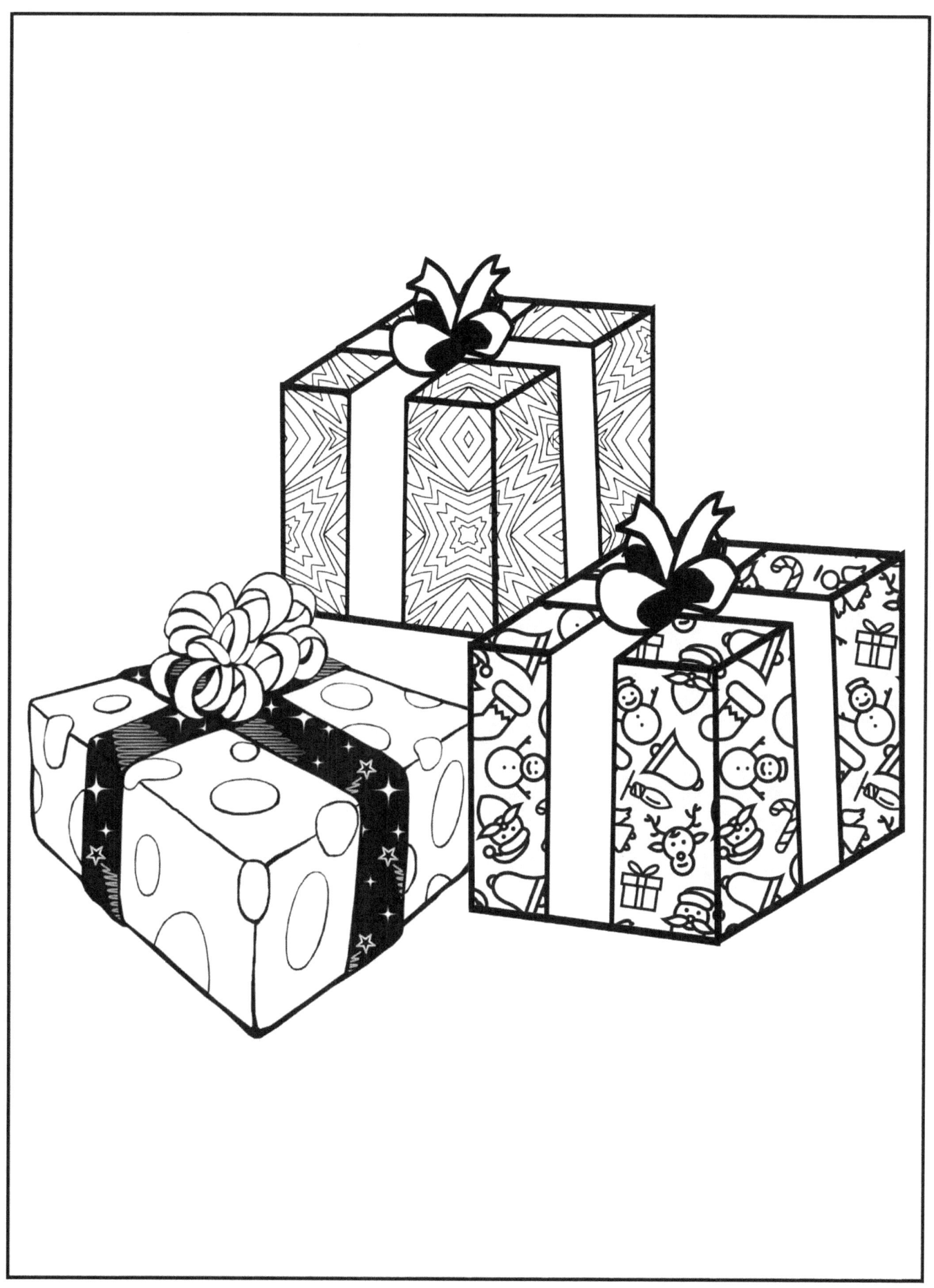

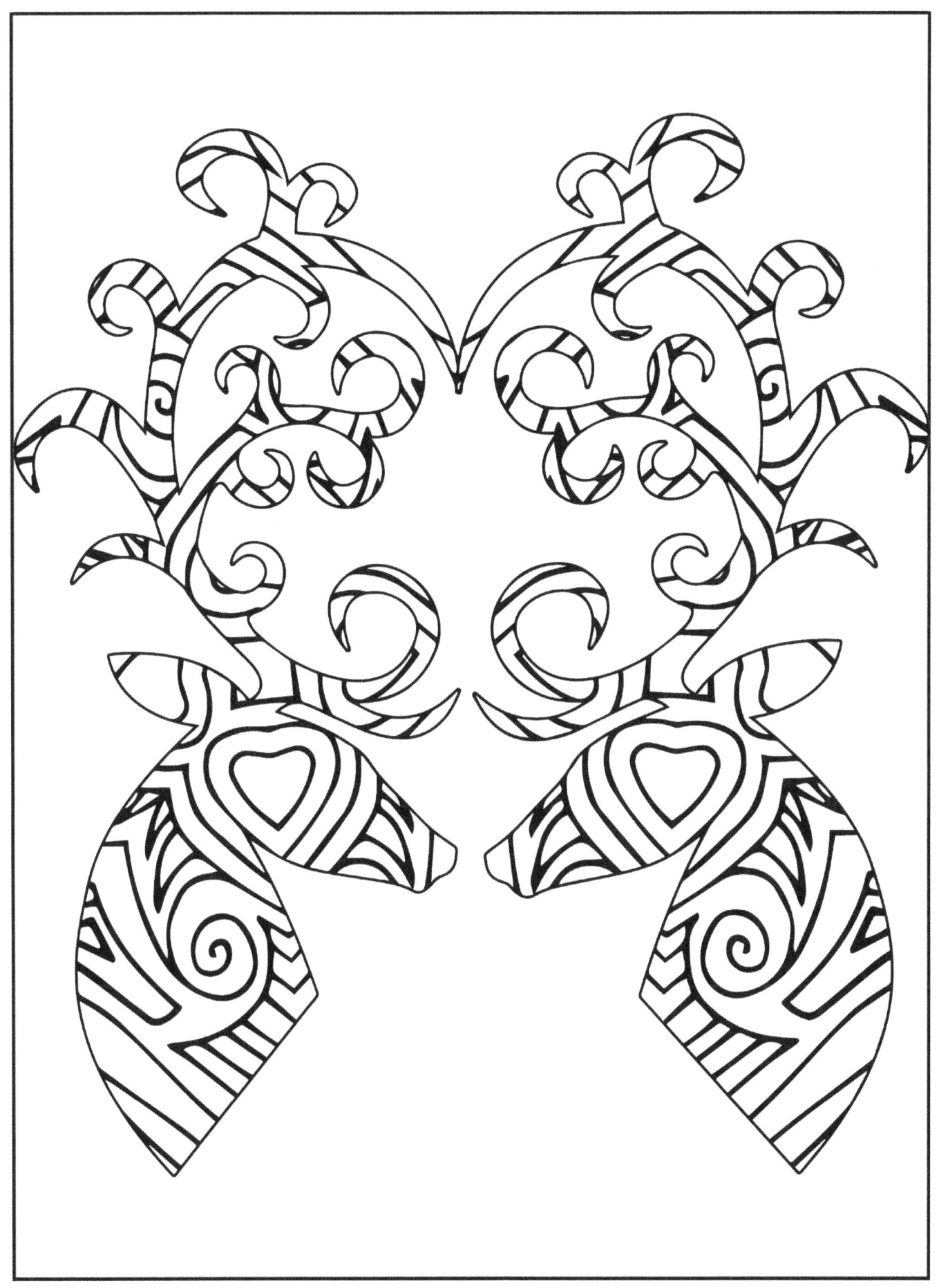

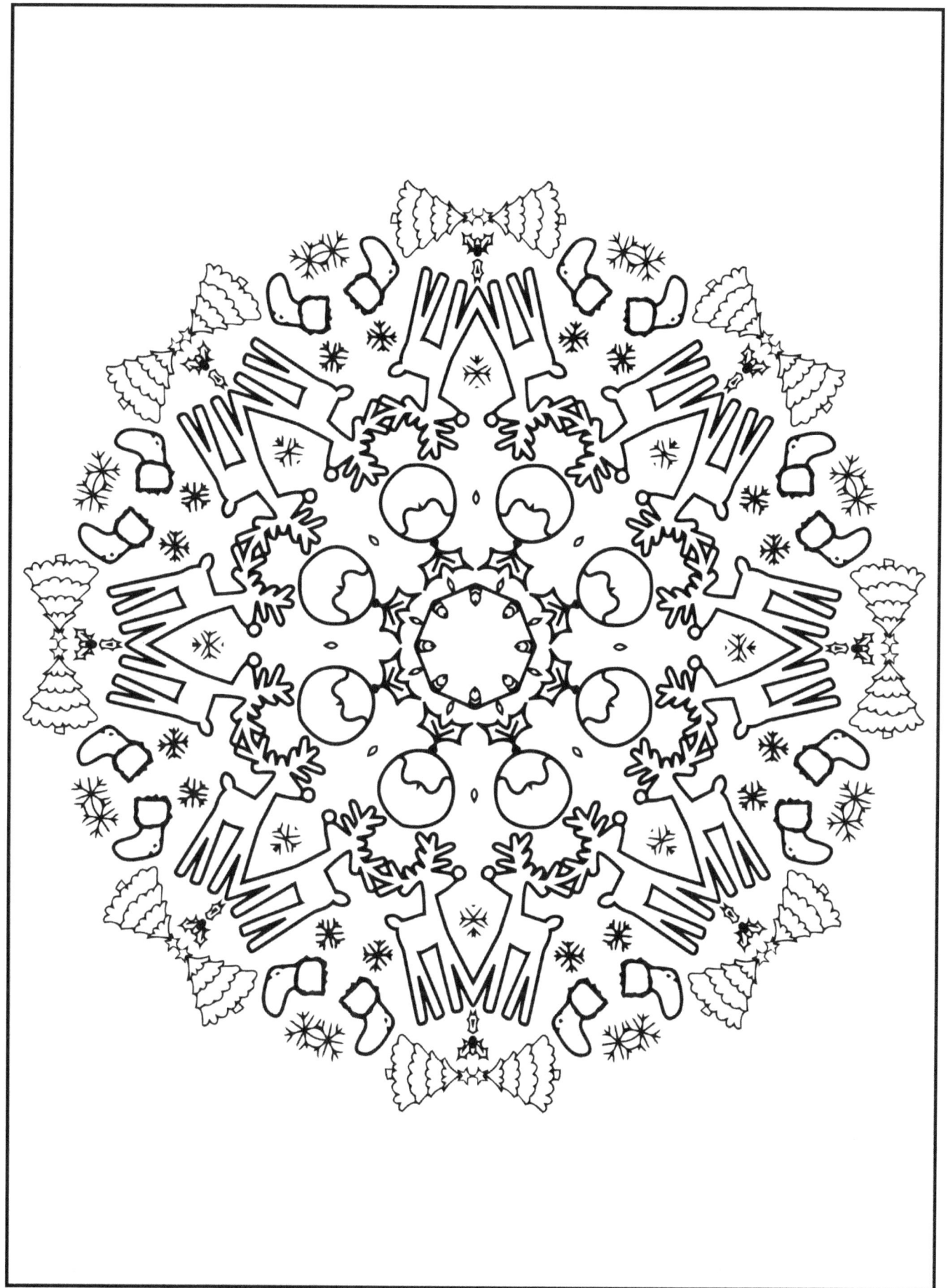

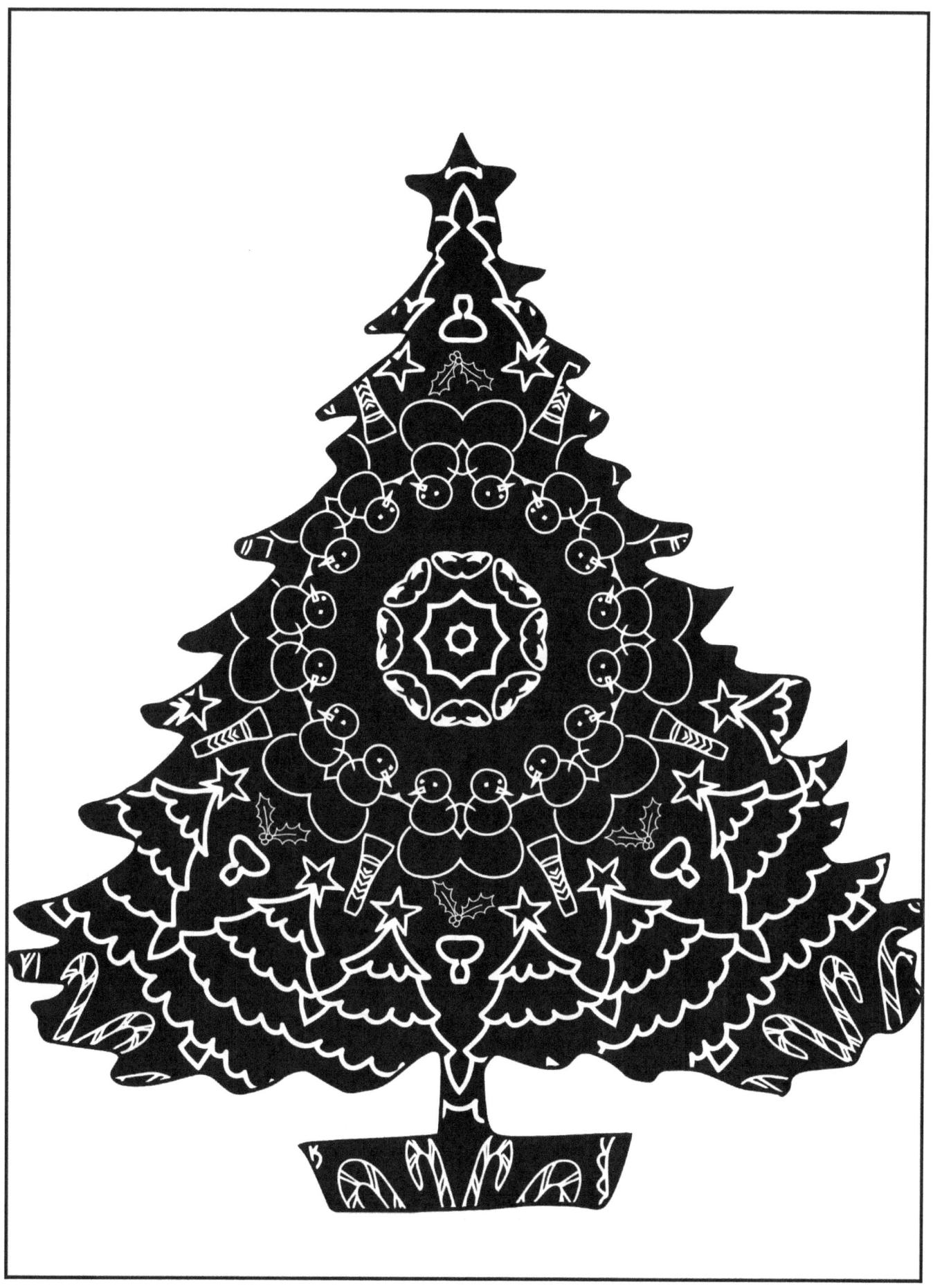

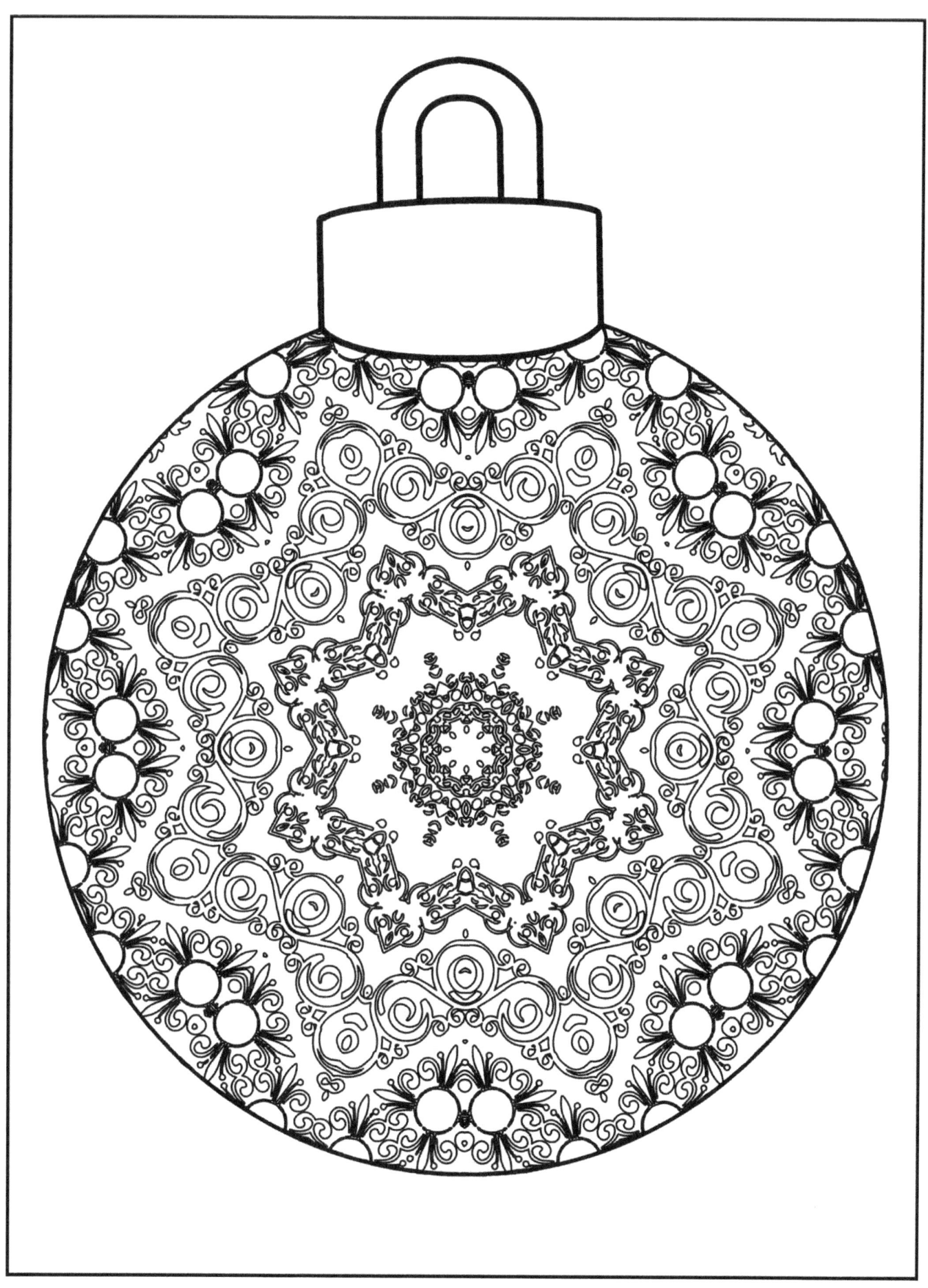

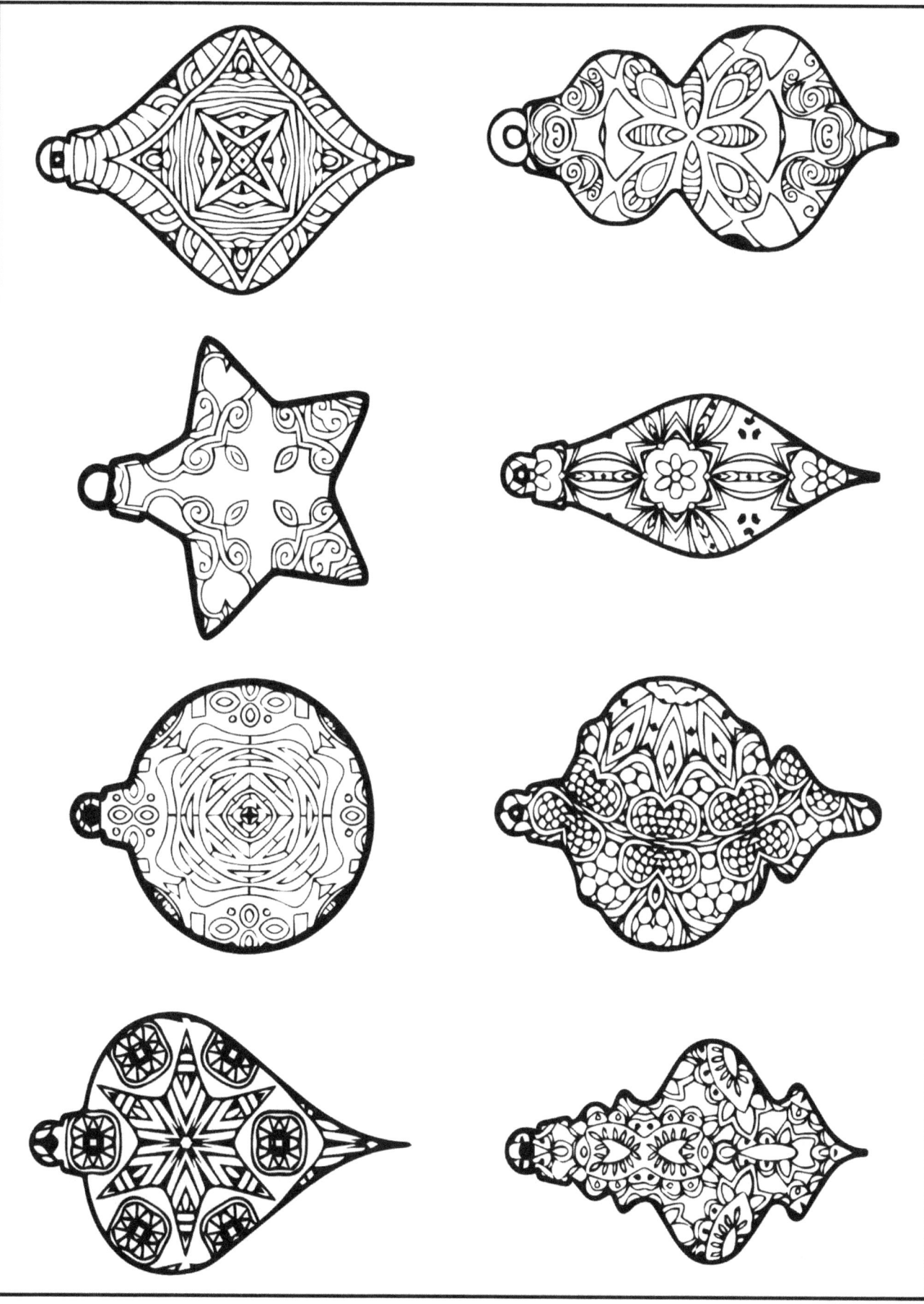

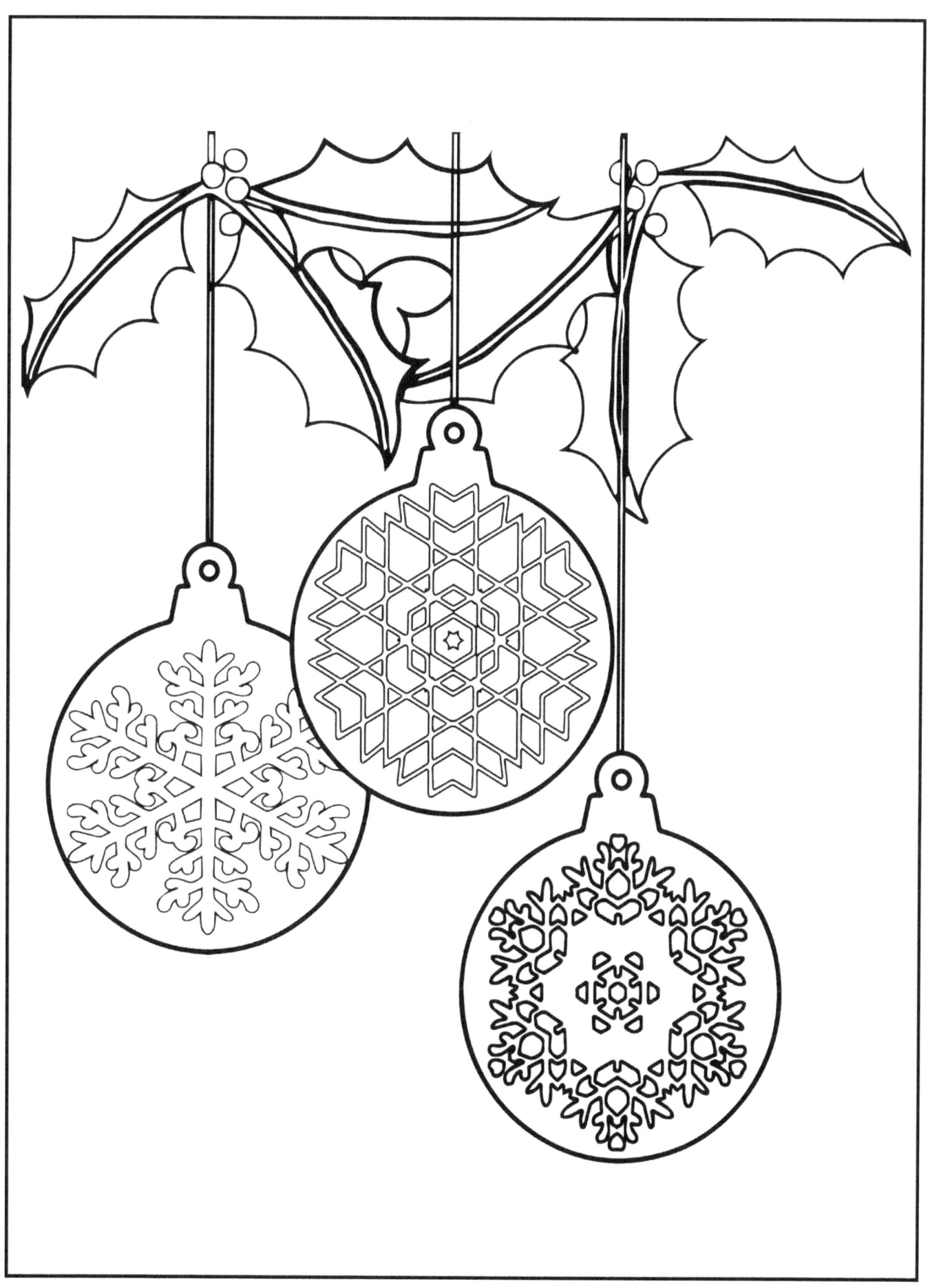

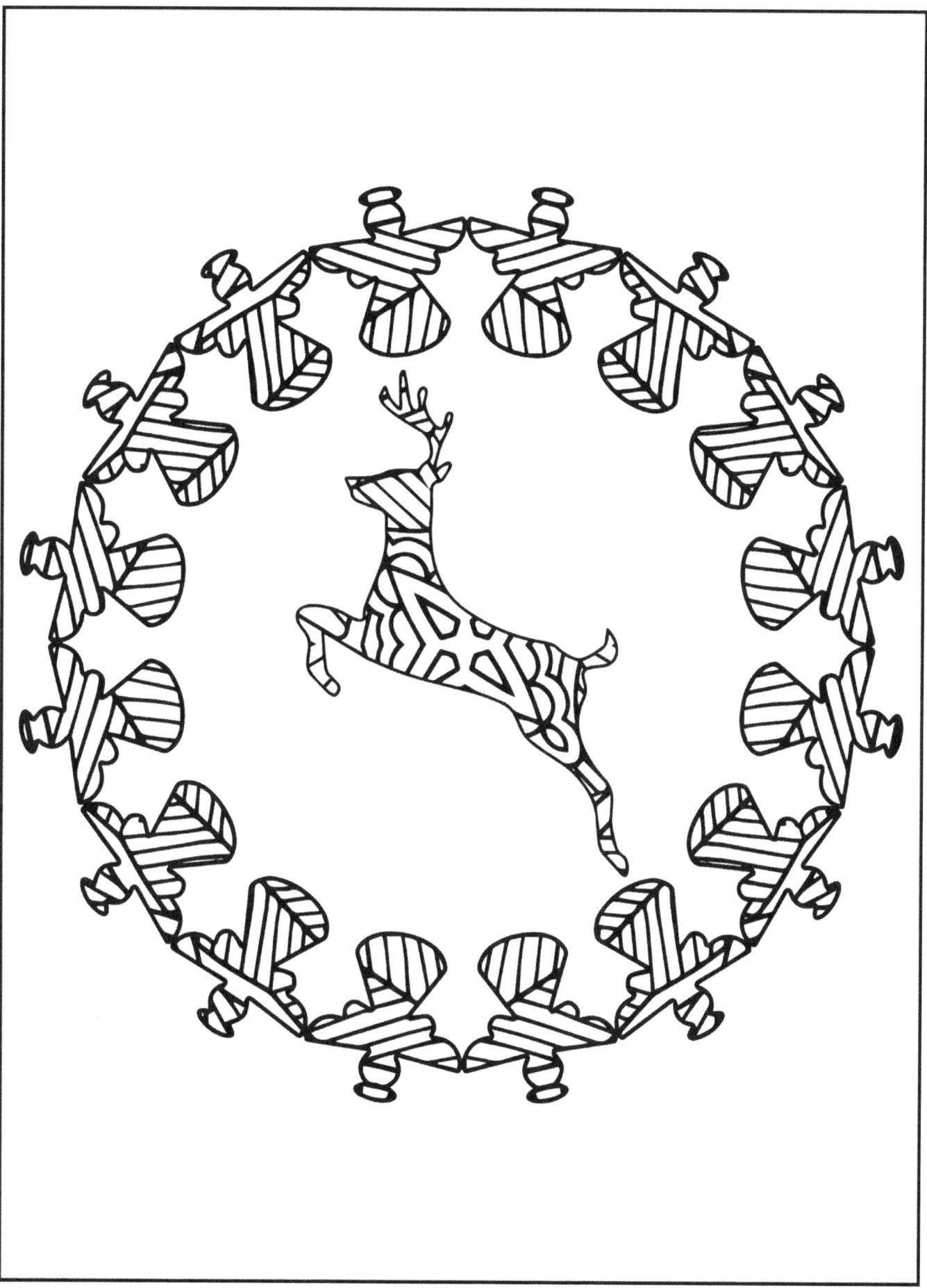

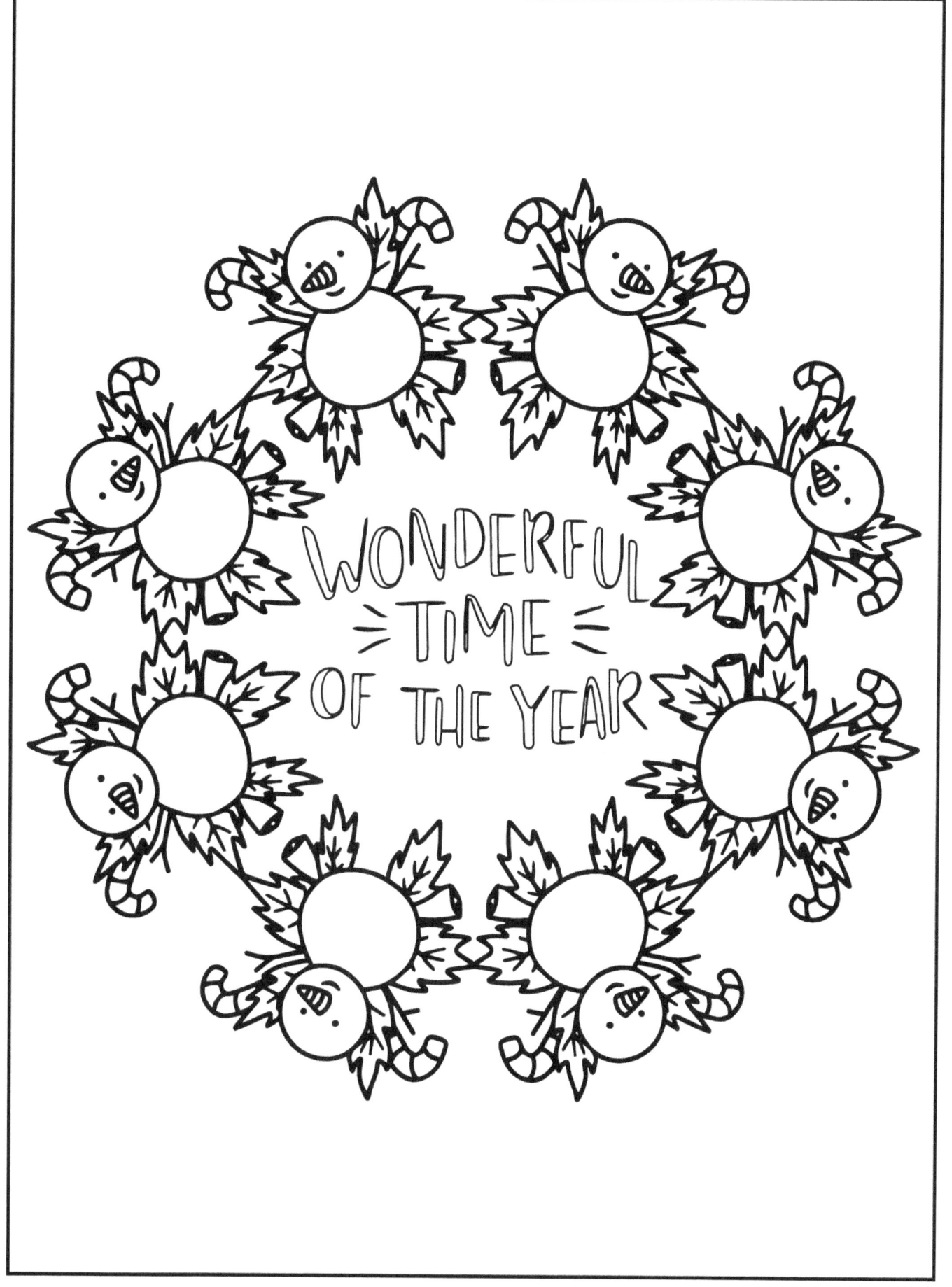

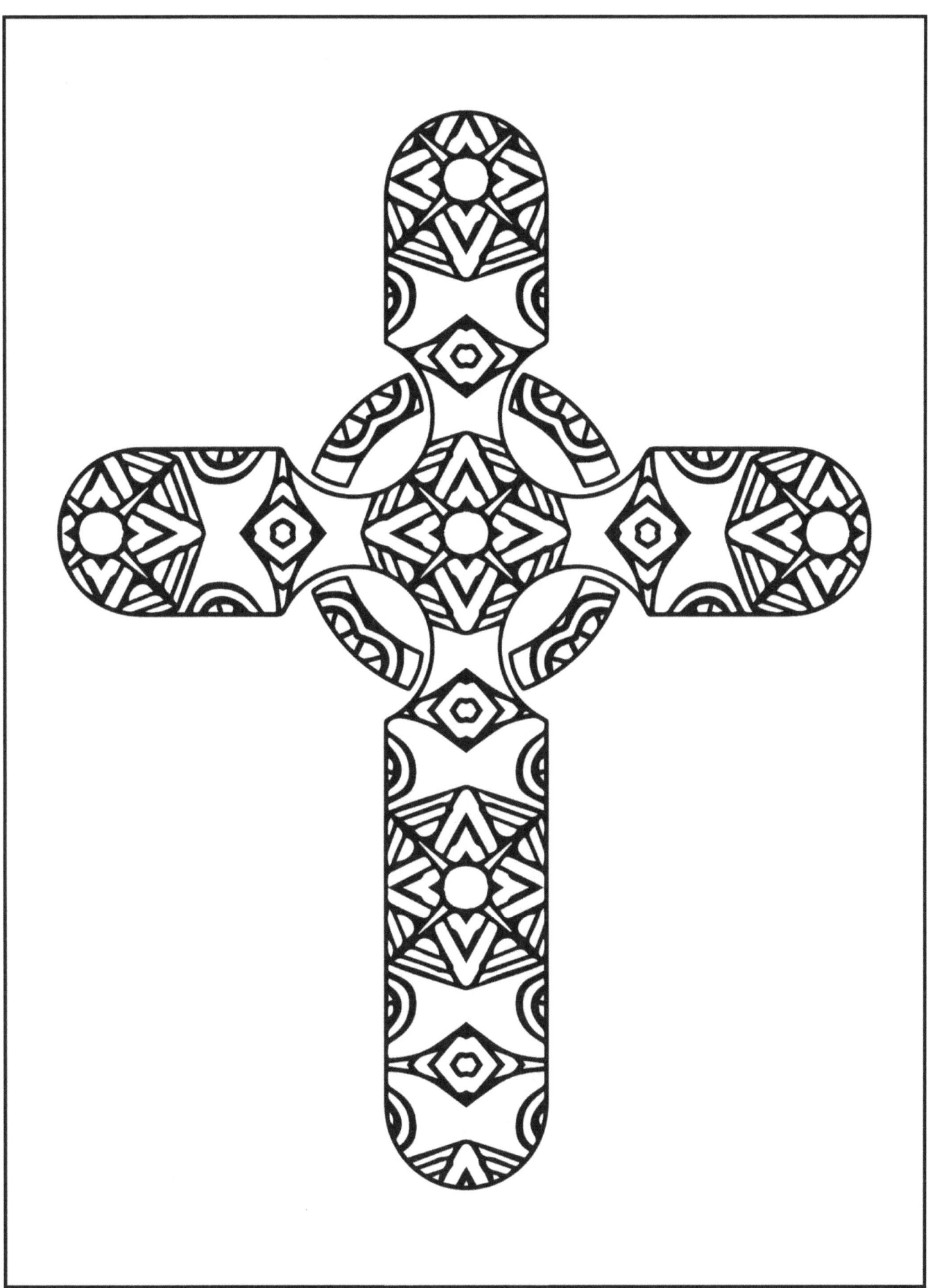

Bonus

Please enjoy these designs from the
Color Your Way To Happy
Series of Adult Coloring Books

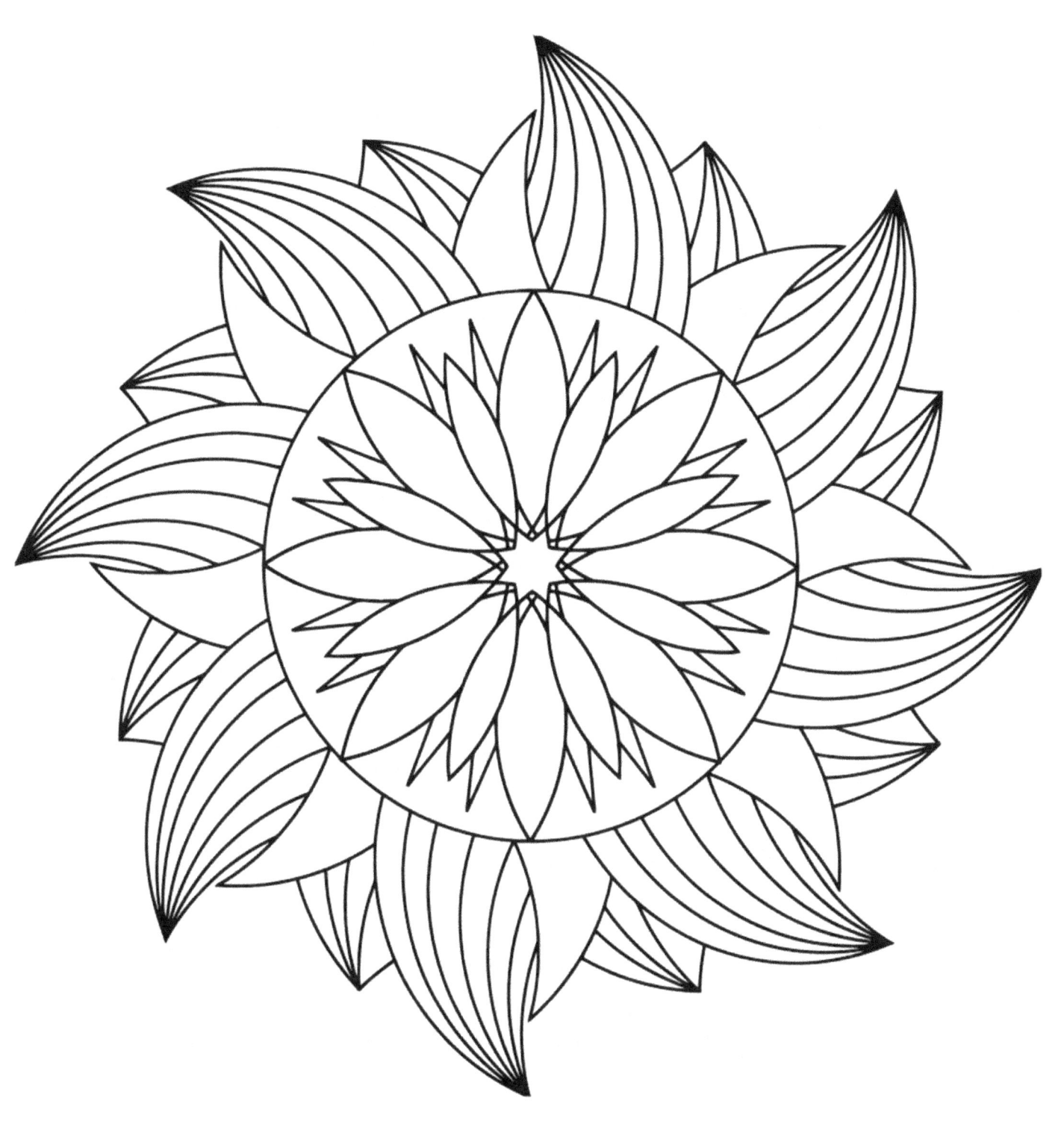

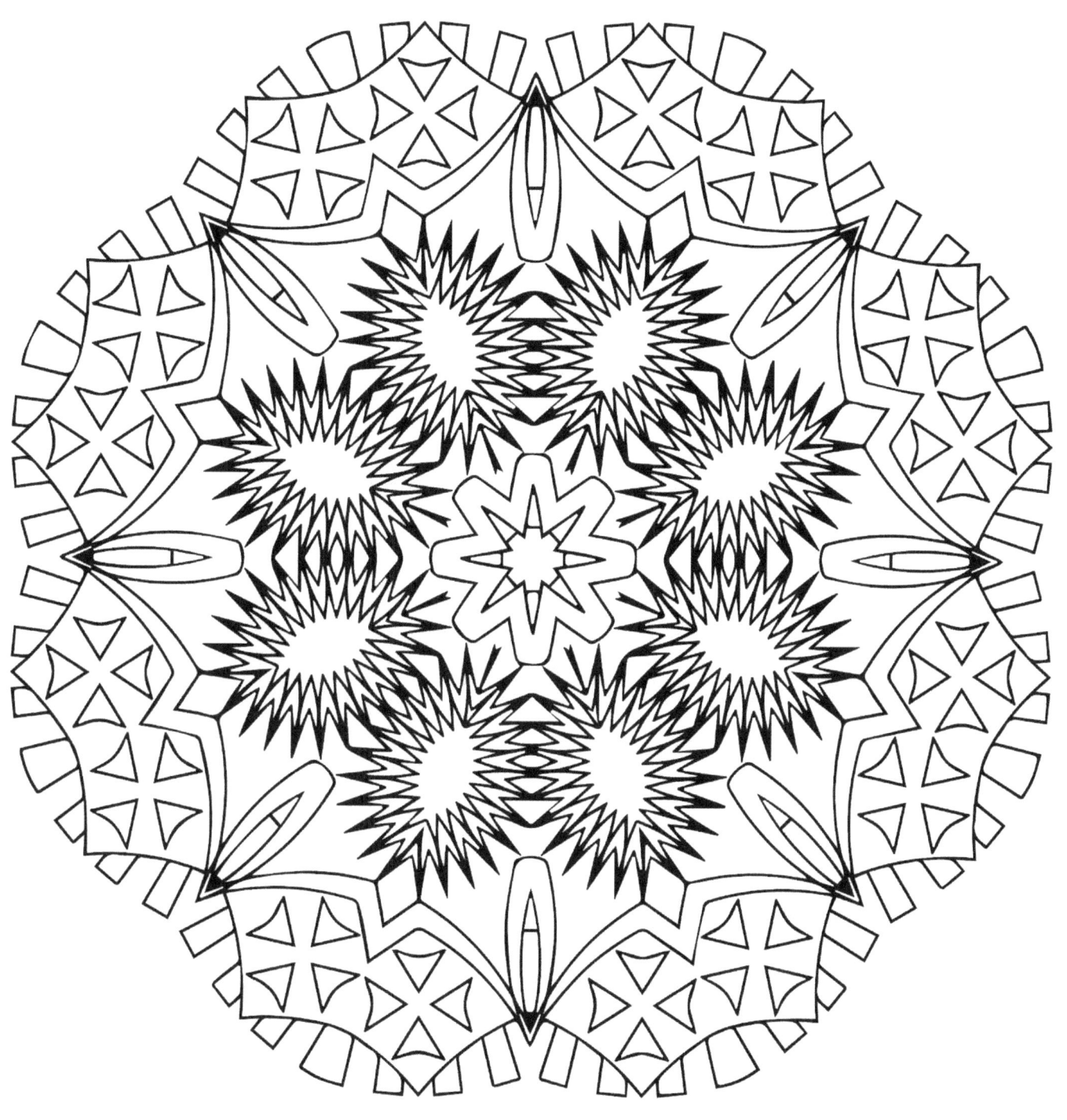

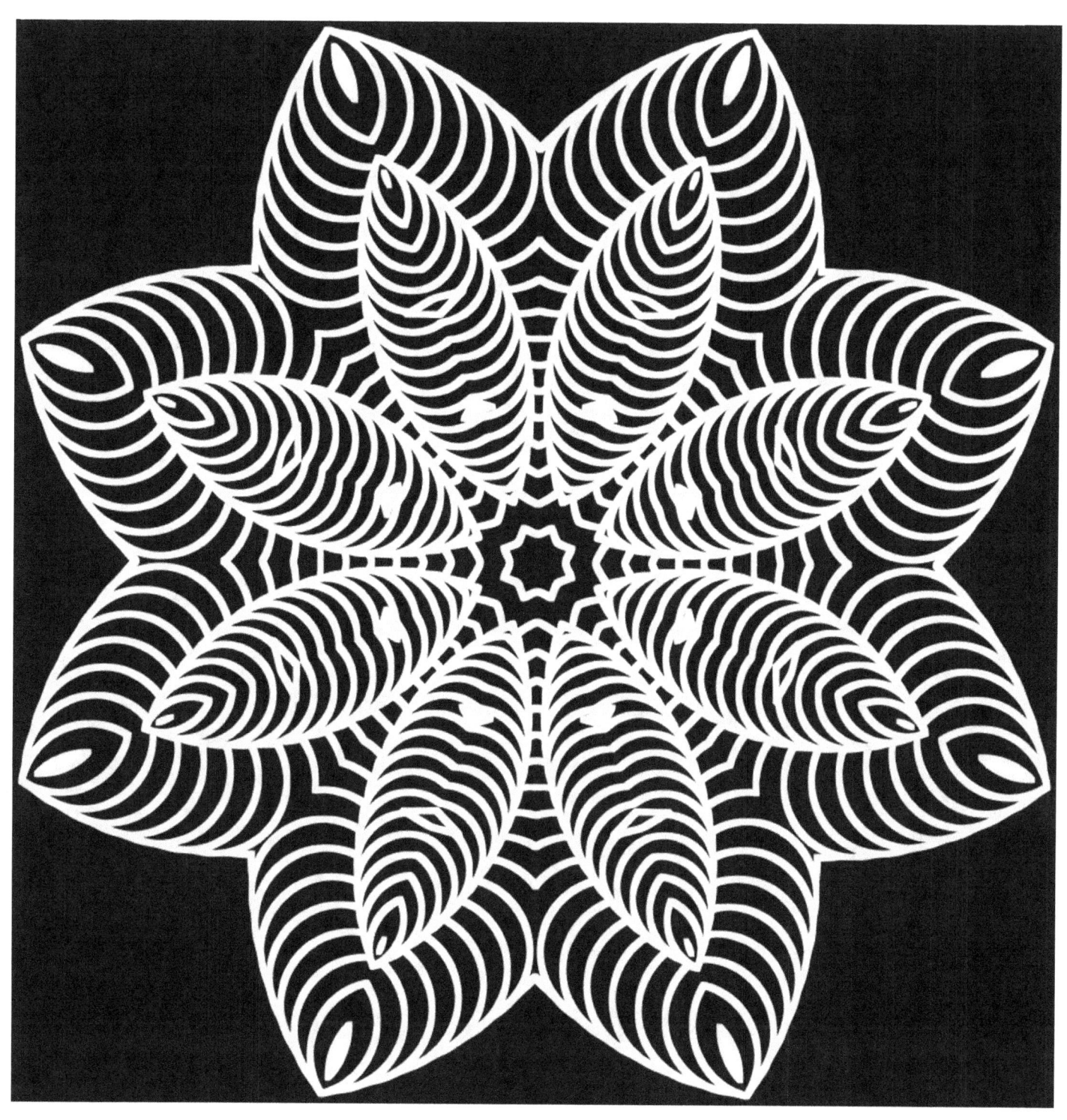

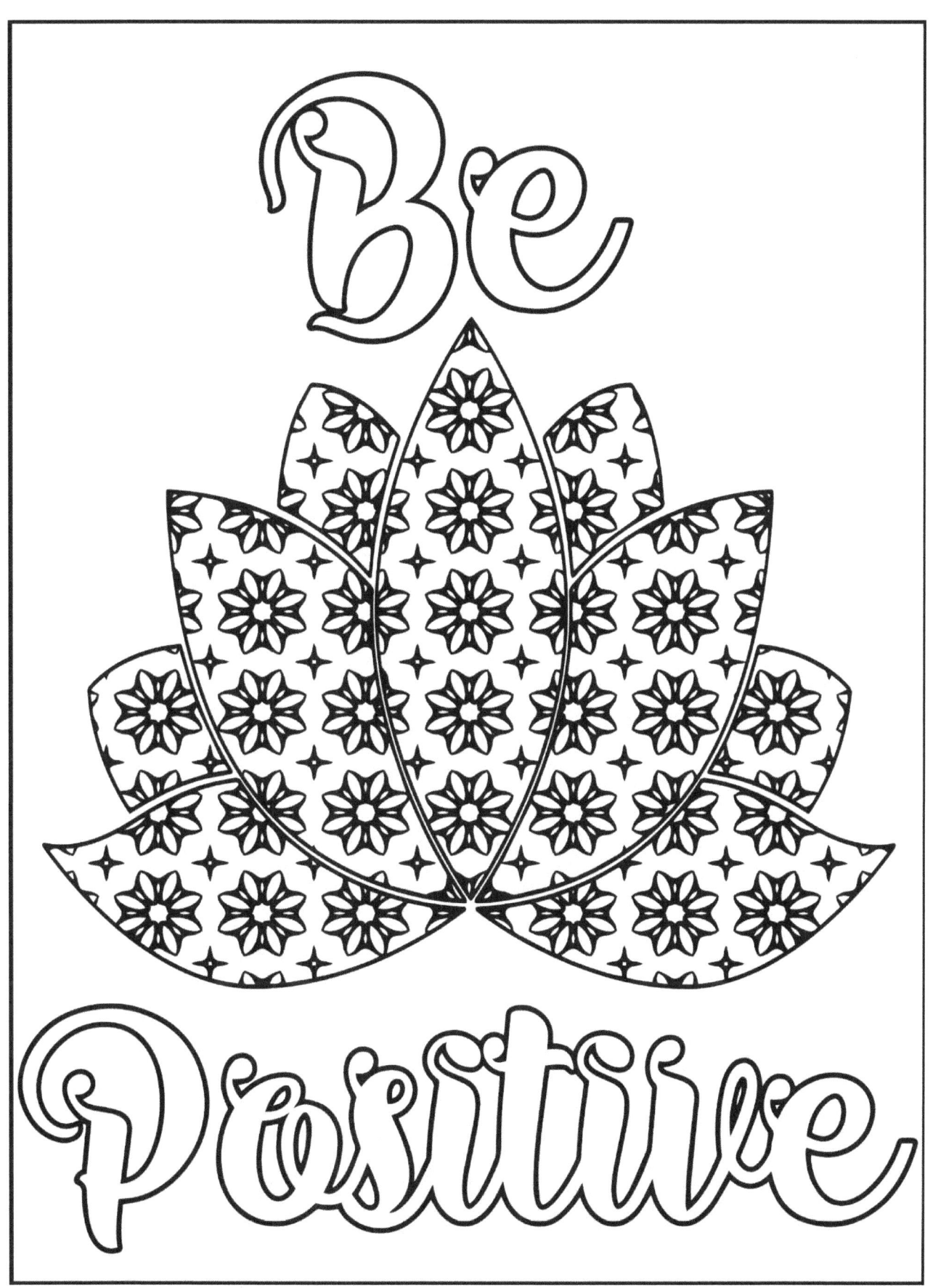

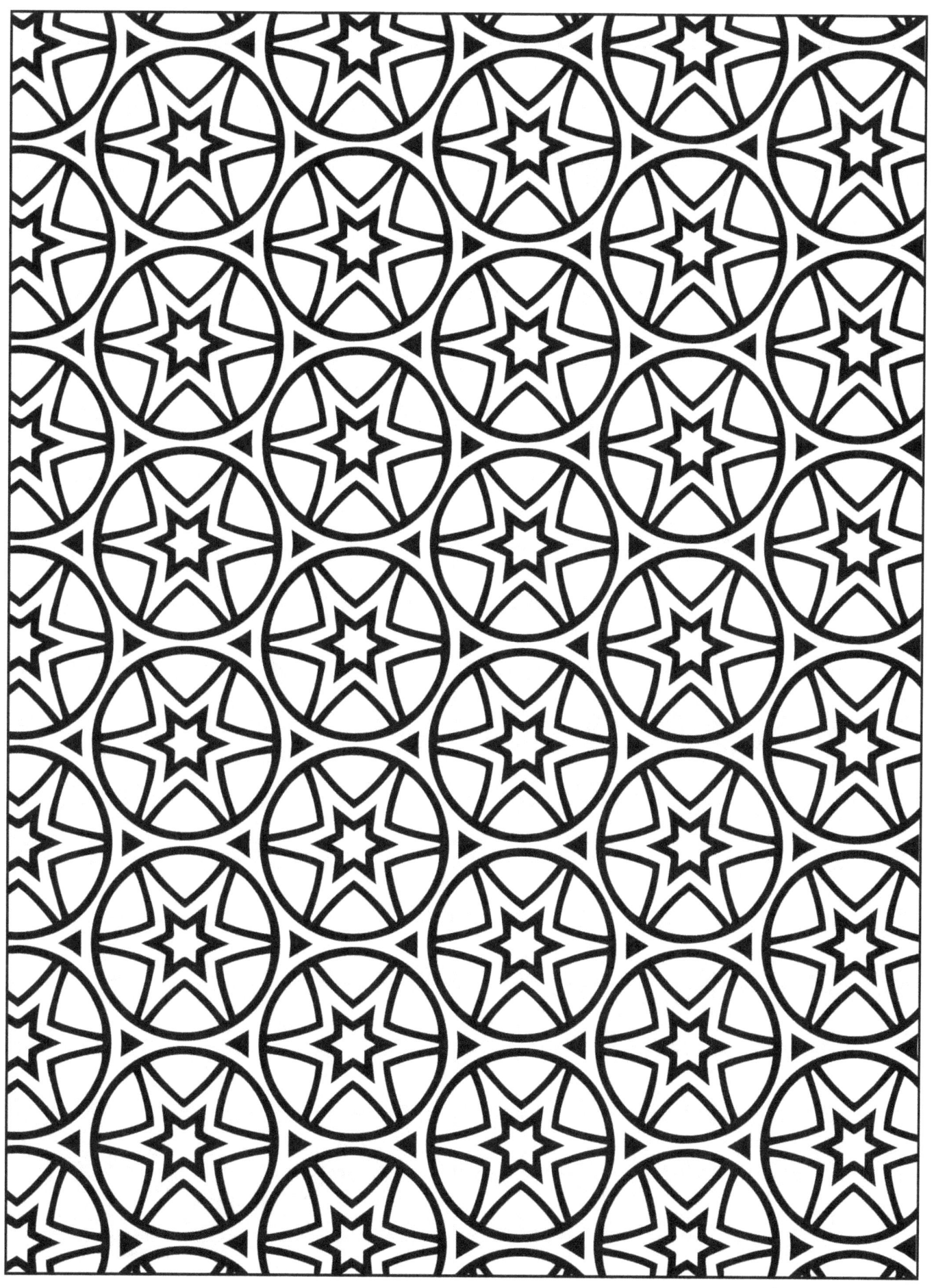

Sample from Patterns for Mindfulness: RELAX Volume 1 © Nerine Martin www.ColorYourWayToHappy.com

Pencils Color Chart

Product Name:

Stay In Touch & Explore More!

If you would like to be kept up-to-date with coloring tips, new book releases and news, and receive a FREE coloring book, please take a moment and visit www.ColorYourWayToHappy.com/freebie and enter your details.

Remember to Like, Share & Comment on my Facebook page and I would love to see some of your finished coloured pages. I encourage you to share them in other Facebook coloring groups and on my page located at **www.facebook.com/ColorYourWayToHappy**

If you post a picture that you've colored from my book, in any Facebook coloring groups, I would really appreciate it if you could please tag me (#ColorYourWayToHappy) in that post and add the name of the book too.

If you've enjoyed coloring my book, would you please leave me a review on Amazon and spread the word to your friends! Your positive review and 5 stars will go a long way to letting other readers know they'll probably like this book too!

All you need to do is type this link into your Internet browser:
http://ColorYourWayToHappy.com/Christmas

Thank you and remember to have fun and *'Color Your Way to Happy'*!

Merry Christmas

Nerine ☺

P.S. Did you know you can also purchase a PDF instant downloadable version to print at home? This is a great way to print your favorite pages as many times as you like, or to print onto cardstock. You can purchase a downloadable version of all my coloring books at a discounted price at **www.ColorYourWayToHappy.com.**

OTHER COLORING BOOKS BY NERINE MARTIN

Mandalas for Mindfulness Volume 1
Mandalas for Mindfulness Volume 2
Neon Mandalas for Mindfulness Volume 3
Patterns for Mindfulness: RELAX Volume 1
Color Your Way Through Anxiety
My Coloring Organizer

You can also find Nerine's designs featured in:
Adult Coloring Book Treasury 1
Adult Coloring Book Treasury 2
(Available from www.Amazon.com)

Share your colored pages from Nerine's books at:
www.facebook.com/ColorYourWayToHappy

The *Color Your Way To Happy* adult coloring book series,
offers you an escape from the daily pressures of life,
to a relaxing state of calm and mindfulness.

Grab your copy today and go 'Color Your Way To Happy'.

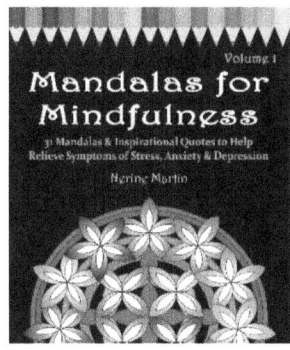 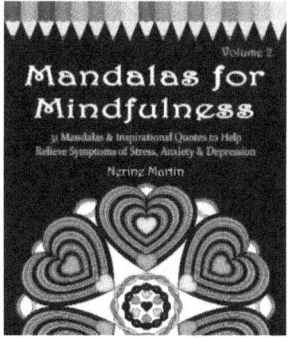 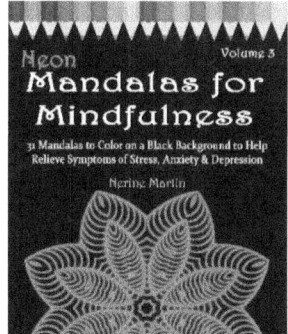
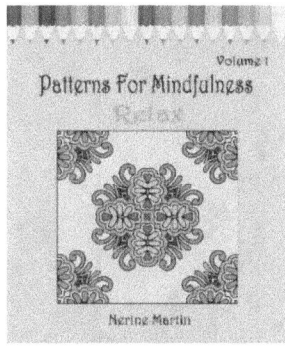 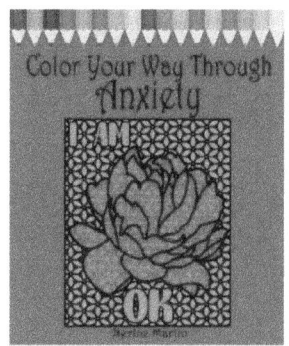 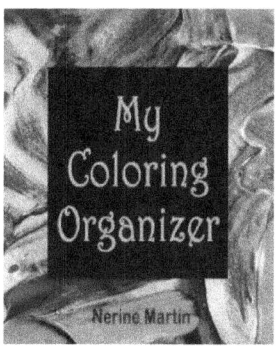

Tear out this blotter page and place behind
the page you are coloring to protect from bleed through ☺

Tear out this blotter page and place behind
the page you are coloring to protect from bleed through ☺